W9-BXU-125

THE UNIVERSITY OF MAINE
AT AUGUSTA

BENNETT D. KATZ LIBRARY

CULTURAL ISSUES IN PLAY THERAPY

CULTURAL ISSUES IN PLAY THERAPY

❧

Edited by

ELIANA GIL
ATHENA A. DREWES

Foreword by Joyce C. Mills

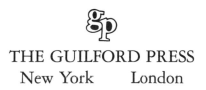

THE GUILFORD PRESS
New York   London

© 2005 The Guilford Press
A Division of Guilford Publications, Inc.
72 Spring Street, New York, NY 10012
www.guilford.com

All rights reserved

No part of this book may be reproduced, translated, stored in a retrieval system, or transmitted, in any form or by any means, electronic, mechanical, photocopying, microfilming, recording, or otherwise, without written permission from the Publisher.

Printed in the United States of America

This book is printed on acid-free paper.

Last digit is print number: 9 8 7 6 5 4 3 2 1

Library of Congress Cataloging-in-Publication Data

Cultural issues in play therapy / edited by Eliana Gil, Athena A. Drewes.
    p. cm.
  Includes bibliographical references and index.
  ISBN 1-59385-012-3 (hardcover)
  1. Play therapy. 2. Play therapy—Cross-cultural studies. I. Gil, Eliana.
II. Drewes, Athena A., 1948–

RJ505.P6C84 2005
618.92'891653—dc22   2004008979

On the seashore of endless worlds the children meet with shouts and dances.
They build their houses with sand and they play with empty shells.
With withered leaves they weave their boats and smilingly float them on the vast
    deep.
Children have their play on the seashore of worlds.

—RABINDRANATH TAGORE

We dedicate this book to the children of the world with whom we work.

About the Editors

Eliana Gil, PhD, RPT-S, ATR, is coordinator of the Abused Children's Treatment Services of Inova Kellar Center, in Fairfax, Virginia. She specializes in the treatment of abused children and their families. Dr. Gil is also director of Starbright Training Institute. She is an adjunct faculty member at Virginia Tech, a registered art therapist, a registered play therapy supervisor, and a licensed marriage and family therapist.

Athena A. Drewes, PsyD, RPT-S, is a licensed psychologist and registered play therapist and supervisor. She is director of Clinical Training and the APA Psychology Doctoral Internship and gives direct service to foster care children and families at The Astor Home for Children in Poughkeepsie, New York. Dr. Drewes has been a play therapist for over 25 years, working with children and adolescents across all types of mental health and school-based settings. She is on the Board of Directors of the Association for Play Therapy, founder and past president of the New York Association for Play Therapy, and Adjunct Professor of Play Therapy at Mount Saint Mary College in Newburgh, New York. Dr. Drewes has written numerous articles on play therapy and coedited a book, *School-Based Play Therapy* (with Lois J. Carey and Charles E. Schaefer, 2001, Wiley).

Contributors

Diana Bermudez, MA, Department of Counseling, Human and Organizational Studies, George Washington University, Washington, DC

Athena A. Drewes, PsyD, RPT-S, The Astor Home for Children, Poughkeepsie, New York

Eliana Gil, PhD, RPT-S, ATR, Abused Children's Treatment Services, Inova Kellar Center, and Starbright Training Institute for Child and Family Play Therapy, Fairfax, Virginia

Geri Glover, PhD, LPCC, NCC, RPT-S, Child and Adolescent Behavioral Health Services, Alamo Navajo Health Clinic, Magdalena, New Mexico

Sonia Hinds, RN, MSN-CS-P, Chesapeake Play Therapy Institute, Chesapeake Beach, Maryland

Silvina Hopkins, MA, LPC, Abused Children's Treatment Services, Inova Kellar Center, Fairfax, Virginia

Virginia Huici, MA, LPC, Abused Children's Treatment Services, Inova Kellar Center, Fairfax, Virginia

Shu-Chen Kao, PhD, Department of Guidance and Counseling, National Chunghua University of Education, Chunghua, Taiwan

Cathy A. Malchiodi, ATR, LPCC, LPAT, REAT, National Institute for Trauma and Loss in Children, Grosse Pointe Woods, MI

Foreword

The weaving of a traditional Navajo rug begins as the weaver shears the sheep, collects plants for dye, dyes the wool, and spins the wool until it becomes yarn. She then finds just the right loom on which to weave her rug. Sitting before it, she sings a prayer song and weaves the pattern that emerges from her heart. All who know about Navajo rugs appreciate their value, strength, spirit, and substance.

It seems to me that Eliana Gil and Athena A. Drewes have metaphorically become weavers in their own right. Instead of yarn, they use cultural knowledge, history, values, and traditions to provide us with a rich compilation of approaches and insights that will enable play therapists to do respectful, sensitive work with culturally diverse children or adolescents and their families. Each chapter is like yarn of a particular color chosen for weaving and must be recognized for the individual brilliance it provides. Woven together, the different chapters create a beautiful pattern . . . a book of substance and heart.

I found myself reading each of the eight comprehensive chapters with enthusiasm and curiosity. (There is also an extremely helpful appendix on multicultural play therapy resources.) The first three chapters, written individually by Eliana (Chapter 1) and Athena (Chapters 2 and 3), expound on moving from sensitivity to competence; the role of play throughout a variety of cultures; and suggestions and research on multicultural play therapy.

In the opening chapter, Eliana begins by sharing the personal insights she has derived from growing up bicultural and highly acculturated in Western culture. She describes the impact of her Ecuadorian heritage and experience, and invites each of us readers to explore our own personal biases, values, and beliefs, and how they can affect and influence the therapeutic relationship. While reading this chapter, I found myself remembering my own issues with being Jewish and how I would often try to hide my Jewishness in a dominant culture in order to be accepted. When someone would find out that I was Jewish and comment, "You don't even look Jewish," I would respond

by saying "Thank you," as if the remark was a compliment. It wasn't until I
was in the center of a violent confrontation in a work environment when I
was 18 years old, and was called "a dirty little Jew," that my heart and spirit
felt a wake-up call to embrace rather than hide who I was.

At the heart of Chapter 1, Eliana shares her view of becoming a cross-
culturally competent therapist as a process that has three distinct levels:
(1) building sensitivity, (2) responsibly obtaining knowledge, and (3) developing active competence. She elucidates each of these levels through a
case example involving an adopted Chinese girl and her new European
American family.

In Chapter 2, Athena addresses "Play in Selected Cultures: Diversity
and Universality." She shows us the effects of culture and tradition on
children's play and imaginative life in many parts of the world. In particular, Athena extensively explores the relationship between play and toys,
the themes of children's play, and parent–child interactions in play within
a variety of cultures.

Athena begins Chapter 3 with a series of very helpful suggestions for
conducting multicultural play therapy. Too often, differences of race, culture, gender, and class are overlooked or actually denied by therapists. I
have often walked into playrooms and have seen only white-faced dolls,
or dolls with dark or brown faces but with "white" features. I have seen
fancy two-story Barbie-like dollhouses in playrooms serving children who
live in small tin-roofed houses or inner-city apartments. We must ask ourselves what kinds of messages children receive in therapeutic environments
where their socioeconomic background or ethnicity is not valued. Athena
then reviews the relatively few studies that have been conducted to date
on cross-cultural play therapy.

In Chapters 4–8, seven highly gifted contributing authors share personal
and professional stories from their own cultural experience, as well as address culture-specific issues that are essential in the field of play therapy.

In Chapter 4, "The Impact of Culture on Art Therapy with Children,"
Cathy A. Malchiodi shares her extensive experience as an art therapist,
describing the numerous considerations therapists need to embrace in order
to provide culturally sensitive art therapy to young clients. These considerations include ethnicity, acculturation, regionalization, socioeconomic
status, gender, and religious or spiritual affiliations.

Sonia Hinds offers an invaluable glimpse into the African American
"village," as she calls it in Chapter 5. Throughout the chapter, she openly
tackles such issues as racism (both in history and in present-day U.S. society), gender, and religion; she also describes valuable interventions, appropriate toys, and creative arts, including music. As she beautifully states,
"To be a true healer to troubled children, it is imperative that the therapist
gain cultural understanding by entering the village in an attempt to learn

the norms, values, customs, and wherever appropriate, weave these into psychotherapeutic interventions."

Silvina Hopkins, Virginia Huici, and Diana Bermudez, all originally from Latin America, provide us with a window into the beliefs, customs, and values inherent in Hispanic families. They help us to see that the pace of therapy must be considered, along with the role played by stereotypes, discrimination, and gender, in the overall treatment and outcome of a therapeutic intervention.

I found Geri Glover's discussion in Chapter 7 of working with Native American children insightful and extremely important for any therapist who may work with this population. With sensitivity, knowledge, and case examples, she highlights the historical trauma Native Americans have experienced since the arrival of Europeans on this continent, as well as the effects of poverty, unemployment, and physical illnesses on this population today. Of equal importance is her appreciation for the traditional values of "generosity, respect for elders, and respect for creation, harmony, and individual freedom."

In Chapter 8, Shu-Chen Kao examines the importance of "Play Therapy with Asian Children." Although she draws to a considerable extent on her personal experience as a Chinese therapist working with children of Chinese (as well as European) descent, she describes four general ethnic groupings within the Asian community: (1) Pacific Islanders; (2) Southeast Asians; (3) East Asians, including Chinese, Japanese, and Koreans; and (4) South Asians, including Indians and Pakistanis. She shares the common threads that run through the cultures, as well as individual differences among the communities, such as background, historical experiences, values, and norms.

In summary, it is clearly time for us as play therapists to recognize that *cultural ecology* must be addressed in order to help families and children heal from such wounds as abuse, domestic violence, fear, pain, grief, or historical trauma. Each author in this book shows us that no simple, universally applicable approach can be used to help children and families of different cultures heal. Each culture must be recognized for its individual history, strengths, and challenges.

And so it is that Eliana Gil and Athena A. Drewes, along with their highly gifted clinician coauthors who have so generously contributed their cultural stories, insights, and concepts, have become modern-day weavers of a metaphorical rug. Like the Navajo rug, this book provides us with a substantive pattern to be treasured, used, and more importantly "lived," as we venture forth in our world of global interconnectedness and heartfelt quest for child and family healing.

JOYCE C. MILLS, PhD

Preface

Eliana Gil: I was raised in Guayaquil, Ecuador, the youngest daughter of Ecuadorian parents who divorced when I was 14. After the divorce, my mother decided to return to the United States, where she had previously lived and worked. Thus, just prior to my 15th birthday (the timing was bad for me because I was mortified to miss my *quincianera*, as I describe in Chapter 1), we moved to Washington, D.C. I had lived in Washington during my second-grade year, when I had had an English immersion experience that was difficult but gave me a solid foundation in the English language. When I came back for eighth grade, I returned to the same small Catholic elementary school to find that I only vaguely remembered one or two of the teachers; however, I was now fairly bilingual, since I had attended a bilingual school in Ecuador. The second time in this school was definitely less stressful in terms of language, but probably a little more challenging in that I was aware of the cultural differences.

Acculturation is quite an experience for anyone; it's compounded for children, whose identity is not quite established and who want desperately to fit into their social group. Therefore, my childhood experiences of traveling back and forth among Washington, New York, Ecuador, and Venezuela were fraught with stressors. I was lucky to have two friends in eighth grade, Joanne and Tracy, who offered me a great deal of warmth and acceptance.

I have been aware of cultural differences all my life because I've lived within, and between, two very different cultures. I know for a fact that I speak and behave differently, depending on where I am and what the social expectations and demands are. At the same time, I've had to dig deep and establish a core sense of who I am and what I can embrace about my native culture—as well as those things I reject, given my opposition to social injustice and racism; my support for gender equality; and my basic interest in humanity and the potential for human connection, regardless of external features.

I grew up in a culture of tremendous class differences, as well as status differences based on color. The poor in Ecuador are very poor, and the rich are beyond wealthy. From the time I was small, I was completely stunned to see these two extremes living side by side. Even when I visited very wealthy homes, I was shocked to see that the helpers (cooks, maids, and nannies) lived in very small rooms off the kitchens with very few comforts.

Probably the most formative experience I had was when I felt true love for one of the children assigned to be my servant. Her name was Chabita, and I've never forgotten her, but I've also never been able to find her as an adult. Chabita was like a sister I didn't have at the time. She and I played for long hours during the day, and at night we shared our deepest secrets. I often sneaked her into my bed, because I couldn't stand her sleeping on the floor next to my bed. She would awaken early in the morning to prepare my breakfast, gather my books, and make sure my uniform was properly pressed. I was mortified when she got in trouble over something she did or didn't do for me. It was very difficult being taught that she was not my friend, only my servant (in other words, she was not someone I was supposed to love). Eventually she was sent away, because there was concern that I had become too attached to her.

For some reason, some of my early family training about social and class distinctions had little influence on me. I rebelled more and more against adhering to social standards about which people I could care about, based on class or the privilege of financial resources. This has remained a constant in my adulthood. I have also noticed that rigid class differentiation seems to be relaxing somewhat in Ecuador, as a new "middle class" seems to be forming there.

At the same time, there are many Ecuadorian values and traditions that I embrace fully, and I've enjoyed working with Hispanics throughout my professional career because I feel a certain connection with them that is inexplicable yet almost tangible to me. Again, I am left respectful of the power of cultural context.

Athena A. Drewes: My maternal grandparents immigrated to the United States from Naxos, Greece. My paternal grandfather immigrated from Hungary, and my paternal grandmother was a second-generation American, with her mother's family having previously immigrated from Ireland. I grew up in a predominantly matriarchial household with a strong Greek heritage. My mother was the first of her siblings to be born in America, while her parents and older siblings were born in Greece. She experienced firsthand what it was like for members of an immigrant family to adjust to America, learn the language, and find jobs beneath the status they were used to in Greece. My mother shared their stories of immigration, the hurdles they had to overcome, and the prejudices they encountered. My mother was also the first in her generation to marry a non-Greek, which was heresy at the time. The recent movie *My Big Fat Greek Wedding* is a fairly accurate reflection of what my parents' courtship and wedding were like. Although the movie tries not to stereotype Greeks, it unfortunately does in some ways; however, it also conveys some of the strong religious beliefs and other traditions and superstitions that run in Greek families.

My father gave up his religious and cultural heritage to convert to Greek Orthodoxy and take on the Greek culture. He suppressed and denied his mother's Irish Catholic and his father's Hungarian Jewish backgrounds. He had already faced prejudice because of being raised Jewish, but looking Irish; in fact, he had legally changed his last name from Bloom (originally Blum) to Drewes (his mother's maiden name), in order to improve his job opportunities and lessen prejudice. He never spoke about his dual heritage or celebrated it. I did not learn the truth of his background until after his death in 1979, when I was an adult.

My family's overt cultural identity was therefore Greek American; the foods, traditions, customs, and superstitions of that culture were embraced and followed. I grew up within the Greek American setting of church and youth groups. Yet I felt like an outsider, since I did not have a Greek last name or speak fluent Greek—both of which were quickly noticed by Greek friends and commented upon. I learned to understand what it was like for some persons to stereotype me on the basis of my culture and unusual first name, and for others to be prejudiced against me because I was not a "pure" Greek. I also came to understand how cultural identity can have a strong impact on a family and its views. In particular, I saw how cultural superstitions can carry significant weight. For instance, I learned how people can be suspicious of obtaining outside help or mental health support, because it was strongly believed that "you do not air your dirty laundry in public" and should keep problems within the family.

Yet I am able as an adult to look back and embrace my ethnic heritage on both sides of my family, and to use this knowledge and experience in my work in cross-cultural play therapy. As noted above, I am particularly sensitized to the fact that some deeply embedded superstitions and beliefs that go beyond the surface religion are passed on culturally within families. These beliefs and superstitions play a strong part in how families function or respond to outside help; as such, they have to be understood, honored, and worked with. Families with strong cultural identities can often be deeply suspicious of clinicians who are trying to be helpful, and of the mental health system in general. However, this may be a "healthy suspicion." As therapists, we may tend to expect clients to be willing to engage in treatment the moment they walk in the door. However, we must have an understanding of the cultural history of racism and prejudice, as well as an understanding of ourselves. We need to use ourselves and our awareness of our own cultural identity in the treatment process, so that it engages clients who are initially hesitant.

In work with a child and family from a different culture, I find it essential to ask during intake or the first session about the family's spiritual supports, its cultural beliefs, and even its basic views of play. It is easy to stereotype another culture on the basis of something we've read or some movies we've seen—or to take the opposite tack of not acknowledging or ignoring the cultural difference, thinking that it doesn't matter. But we must avoid this by keeping dialogue open with families. We need to look at the members of each family as distinct individuals, and to adjust our clinical lens for each new family. After the first generation in America, it can be hard to tell what cultural background a person has or identifies with. The sense of cultural identity, and the reactions this produces, will differ for each person. We must not be shy or hesitant to ask.

My 10 years of working in a residential treatment center with severely emotionally disturbed children ages 5–12 years, of diverse races/ethnicities, religions, and national origins, have taught me a lot. I had to overcome my reluctance to ask children, staff, and families directly about the cultural traditions they followed; the cultural games they played; and their clothing, hairstyle, and food preferences. We all have to overcome our tendency to avoid offending others and our subsequent reluctance to ask such questions, in order to learn about and engage in others' cultures and thus to become effective cross-cultural play therapists.

Both of us: Play therapists are in a unique position to do effective cross-cultural work with children and families. Play therapists are less entrenched in verbal communication than other types of therapists usually are; they create opportunities for symbolic exchange of ideas; and they value the use of fantasy, pretending, imagery, storytelling, and metaphors. Play therapists are also much more interested in children as individuals than in their "problem behaviors." Those behaviors are usually viewed as forms of "acting out" that communicate underlying aspects of self. All these characteristics are conducive to success in cross-cultural treatment.

In order to work effectively with children of various cultures, it is important for play therapists to collect toys and other materials that will give these children the chance to explore, talk, solve problems, abreact, or project their inner worlds. Play therapists must also maintain a contextual approach to treatment—one that takes into account each child's and family's indigenous culture, degree of acculturation to the new culture, and adjustment to social demands and expectations, along with any cultural schisms within the family. Finally, it is important for play therapists to make learning about different cultures a continuing process, and to reevaluate and adjust their approaches to practice accordingly, so that their playrooms will be both welcoming and therapeutic for multicultural clients.

This book is in no way a comprehensive or final view of cross-cultural work in play therapy. It is, however, a first step in assisting play therapists on the journey to becoming cross-culturally competent. The chapter authors have all undertaken a personal exploration of their work in order to provide professional guidelines that will encourage our thinking in this area. Although the chapters were written independently of each other, the similarities in process and outcome are striking. All the authors draw on their own cultural identities as a framework for describing how to provide a therapeutic context for children that honors *their* cultural identities. The guidelines range from very concrete to more abstract encouragement for developing a commitment to professional growth in this area. It is our hope that these readings will stimulate introspection and result in a better informed and clear path of action.

ELIANA GIL
ATHENA A. DREWES

Acknowledgments

Eliana Gil: This book was completed during a very difficult period in my life, involving a medical crisis in my family. Luckily, we had a positive outcome. However, I spent 2 months out of the country, which caused many delays for this book.

I want to thank Athena Drewes, who took the lead and bore the brunt of this work, and who provided amazing support for me with her patience and willingness to help me in whatever way I needed. She truly held this project in her heart and mind, and without her it would not have been completed. Athena had contacted me when she asked Charles Schaefer about this topic area and expressed an interest in writing something on the subject. I had likewise talked to Charlie about writing something a few years back, and had not yet had the time to do so. When Athena contacted me, we forged a firm partnership that has fueled our mutual interests. I cannot say in words how much she has inspired me and helped me through this difficult time. I am proud to be associated with her and with this project, and I am profoundly in debt to her for her leadership and kindness to me.

Thanks as always to Rochelle Serwator and The Guilford Press for their ultimate confidence in me, understanding, and sensitivity. I thoroughly enjoy my ideal working relationship with Rochelle and other Guilford Press personnel, and I value it greatly.

Athena A. Drewes: I would especially like to thank Denise Garofalo, head librarian of The Astor Home for Children, Poughkeepsie, New York (a large multiservice mental health facility serving three counties in New York). Denise was relentless in tracking down and obtaining the many necessary research articles and books for my chapters. I am deeply indebted to her. Special thanks to my husband, James R. Bridges, and my sons, Scott Richard

Drewes Bridges and Seth Andrew Bridges, for their support and encouragement. Special thanks also to the Diversity Committee of the Association for Play Therapy (APT) and to APT's membership, who identified the need for this book and in turn encouraged us to write it. Finally, my special, heartfelt thanks to Eliana Gil for her faith in me. It has been a great collaboration!

Contents

PART I

Background and General Considerations

1

❧

From Sensitivity to Competence in Working across Cultures

ELIANA GIL

> I have always felt that the action most worth watching is not at the
> center of things but where edges meet. I like shorelines, weather fronts,
> international borders. There are interesting frictions and incongruities
> in these places, and often, if you stand at the point of tangency, you
> can see both sides better than if you were in the middle of either one.
> This is especially true, I think, when the apposition is cultural.
> —ANNE FADIMAN, *The Spirit Catches You and You Fall Down*
> (1997, p. x)

Ahnna was adopted at the age of 4½ from an orphanage in China. Her
history prior to that age was virtually unknown, except that her mother
had died during childbirth and her birth father was unable and unwilling
to care for her (he apparently held the infant responsible for his wife's
untimely death). Uncharacteristically, a grief-stricken extended family was
not available to raise Ahnna. The maternal grandmother was widowed and
had cared for Ahnna from infancy until 1½ years of age. When Ahnna's
grandmother died, of lymphatic cancer, the father had remarried, and his
wife had just given birth to a son. Ahnna's father remained unwilling to
provide her with a home, and thus Ahnna was placed in the orphanage.

Ahnna was brought to the United States by her adoptive parents, Scott
and Joelle, who had gone through years of infertility treatment and had
waited to adopt a child for over 3 years. Scott and Joelle were college sweet-
hearts and had both been raised in the Midwest. When Scott secured a

position with a national high-tech company, he and his wife relocated to the East Coast. They quickly discovered that the metropolitan area in which they had settled was very fast-paced, and they were homesick for their families. They planned to return to their home state as soon as Scott could establish a good work record, save money, and find another work position closer to home. They traveled to China with great anticipation and chose Ahnna due to her compliant behavior in the orphanage, as well as her "sweet appearance."

A few months after the adoption, Scott and Joelle brought Ahnna to therapy because she was smearing feces, wetting the bed at night, hitting other children in kindergarten, whining and complaining of stomachaches, and becoming aggressive with the family dog. Ahnna was also masturbating in her bed, distressing both her parents, who panicked that this suggested that Ahnna had been sexually abused. They were distraught, weary, and desperate. Their dreams of a happy family had dissipated into a sea of distress. Although they had anticipated some difficulties with the child, they were shocked and somewhat disgusted with Ahnna's behavior. Their expectations were gravely challenged, and they felt incompetent and ashamed.

A number of issues are highlighted in this case, to which I return later in this chapter.

CHANGING VIEWS OF WORKING ACROSS CULTURES

When I first started taking courses on "cultural issues" in the 1970s, there was a predictable and exclusionary focus on ethnicity. Most conferences and workshops that I attended utilized a panel format in which individuals from different ethnicities would speak about their particular ethnic groups. I clearly remember that the speakers would offer similar introductory statements and emphasize the limitations of their presentations. In fact, it was made resoundingly clear that each individual could only speak to his or her experience within a specific ethnic group or culture, and all speakers took great caution not to generalize. Inevitably, audience members left with a perception that they had been trained in cross-cultural sensitivity, when in fact they had been exposed to an extraordinarily narrow view of culture.

This approach was used in the literature as well, and more and more information appeared about specific ethnic groups (Boyd-Franklin, 1989; Falicov, 1998; Gopaul-McNicol, 1993; Koss-Chioino & Vargas, 1999; Sue & Morishima, 1982; Uba, 1994). This was a worthwhile and important first step, in that it allowed readers to become familiar with rather global aspects of cultural diversity. However, as McGoldrick (1998) states emphatically, "theoretical discussions about the importance of ethnicity are practically useless . . . as are 'cookbook' formulations" (p. 22). She cautions that the systematic integration of material on ethnicity in any mental health professional training "remains a 'special issue,' taught at the periphery of psychotherapy training and rarely written about or recognized as crucial by therapists of the dominant groups" (p. 5).

Over time, more sophisticated debate has resulted in careful consideration and discussion of how mental health professionals and others who provide service delivery to the general public can become more sensitive and indeed more responsible in their interactions with clients or patients of different cultural backgrounds. Numerous books on working cross-culturally have enriched the literature with various philosophical, political, and social approaches (Carter, 1995; Lee, 1997, 1999; McAdoo, 1993; Paniagua, 1994; Pinderhughes, 1989; Tseng & Hsu, 1991). Recent efforts seek to examine and ponder the issues in our contemporary context, and advocate more action to demonstrate increased awareness and expressed good intentions (Mason & Sawyerr, 2002; McGoldrick, 1998). Fewer books have focused on cross-cultural work with children (Canino & Spurlock, 2000; Gibbs, Huang, & Associates, 1998; Webb, 2001).

Historically, this issue has not been embraced easily. Many of my colleagues initially resisted cross-cultural training, stating that the training was irrelevant because "I don't do that kind of work. . . . I don't see minority groups in my agency or practice." Allen and Majidi-Ahi (1998) note that "on the therapist's part, there may be a tendency either to deny that race is an issue in the interaction [with clients] or to overcompensate by attributing all of the client's problems to cultural and racial conflict" (p. 153).

The current climate of acknowledged deficits and a move toward the development of cross-cultural competence reflects the need to take more concrete action, and to remain vigilant to many therapists' resistance to and discomfort with integrating cross-cultural thought and action into their service delivery. There is a consensus that a first step in becoming cross-culturally competent is for a therapist to develop an understanding of his or her own ethnic identity and cultural values. McGoldrick (1998) states, "We are all migrants, moving between our ancestors' traditions, the worlds we inhabit, and the world we will leave to those who come after us. For most of us, finding out who we are means putting together a unique internal combination of cultural identities" (p. 8).

It has become clearer and clearer over time that reading about different cultures is not sufficient to elicit a change in behavior (in either therapists or clients), and it is irresponsible to believe that service delivery does not need to shift or expand in order to be effective with diverse populations.

THE EXPANDING DEFINITION
OF "CULTURE" AND ITS IMPLICATIONS
FOR TREATMENT

Falicov (1998) has best defined a broader view of "culture": "Culture is those sets of shared world views, meanings, and adaptive behaviors derived from simultaneous membership and participation in a variety of contexts, such as language; rural, urban, or suburban settings; race, ethnicity, and socioeconomic status; age, gender, religion, nationality; employment, education, and occupation; political ideology; stage of acculturation" (p. 14). Within this context, attention to culture occurs in all service delivery situations.

Certain issues have been articulated as critical in the provision of cross-cultural treatment. Giordano and Giordano (1995) provide the following key organizing guidelines for therapists:

- Assess the importance of ethnicity to patients and families.
- Validate and strengthen ethnic identity.
- Be aware of and use clients' support systems.
- Serve as a "cultural broker."
- Be aware of "cultural camouflage."
- Know that there are advantages and disadvantages in being of the same ethnic group as a client.
- Don't feel you have to "know everything" about other ethnic groups.
- Try to think in categories that allow at least three possibilities.

Other authors have highlighted additional salient issues. Ramirez (1998) discusses personal distance, self-disclosure, and the process of entering treatment as critical concerns for culturally competent therapists. Gibbs and colleagues (1998) note that research has identified many client variables as relevant to cross-cultural therapy—for example, "attitudes toward mental health and mental illness; belief systems about the causes of mental illness and dysfunctional behavior; differential symptomatology, defensive patterns, and coping strategies; help-seeking behaviors; utilization of services; and responsiveness to treatment" (p. 8). Inclan and Herron (1998) underscore the importance of delving into such issues as immigrant status, poverty (and socioeconomic strata in general), status changes, and generational issues. In addition, LaFromboise and Graff Low (1998) point to the need for cross-cultural therapists to make decisions about collaborating with traditional healers and evaluating their clients' desire for "ceremonial healing" (p. 133).

McGoldrick (1998) defines ethnically self-aware and sensitive therapists as those who "achieve a multiethnic perspective, which is open to understanding values that differ from their own, and no longer need to convert others or give up their own values" (p. 22). An emphasis on the building of *competence* and self-evaluation (with training programs taking the lead) appears to be emerging as this field of study continues to evolve across disciplines (Lu, Lum, & Chen, 2001; Roysircar, Sandhu, & Bibbins, 2003; Zimmerman, 2001).

FROM BUILDING SENSITIVITY TO OBTAINING KNOWLEDGE RESPONSIBLY TO DEVELOPING ACTIVE COMPETENCE

When mental health professionals ponder the daunting task of becoming cross-culturally competent, a number of steps must be taken for optimal outcomes. I view this process as involving three distinct levels of response that build upon each other. In my experience, some therapists fall short of the desired outcome because they achieve the first or second level of response independently of the other two.

Building Sensitivity

Building sensitivity entails introspection and a focus of attention on the interactions between self and others. Most training programs set a foundation for cross-cultural sensitivity by inviting students to explore their own cultural and ethnic identification. Being aware of one's own biases and values will assist in the recognition of client issues in this arena. Making sure that the topic is acknowledged and discussed in one's personal and professional life is also critical, in that it creates conscious attention to this topic. Books that stimulate thinking and discussion in this area are highly recommended and contribute greatly to developing ongoing awareness and sensitivity (Tatum, 1997; Webb, 2001).

I am fully bicultural, with high acculturation in both my cultures. As I have described in the Preface to this book, I moved to the United States from Ecuador full time when I was 14 years old. It was especially distressing to me that my *quincianera* (a ritual dance/party given for girls in many Hispanic cultures when they reach age 15) was an experience I would miss, after years and years of anticipating this rite of passage. My acculturation caused great family rifts, and my mother's overprotection and mistrust are still palpable when I think back to my teenage years. I know that working with Hispanic youth is a challenge for me, since I tend to sympathize (non-systemically) with the plight of bicultural youth. At the same time, I learned many heroic values from my parents, especially my mother, who brought her children to a new country to offer them a better education and more opportunities. As I prepared to meet Ahnna, I thought about my own journey here (albeit at a much older age) and the difficulties and rewards of acculturation. I also recognized my hesitation in working with parents of a bicultural child. I worked hard at self-evaluation during treatment with this family, understanding well that my own identity as bicultural would affect how I viewed this child and family. I decided to forgo a set agenda, but rather to continue interacting with Ahnna and her parents, learning about myself and sharing aspects of myself as the therapy progressed.

There are numerous ways of becoming sensitized to (or sensitive of) others' plight. The most obvious way is to empathize with other persons by trying to understand their experiences, their struggles, their resources, and motivations. This is easier said than done, and it is a step that is often skipped partially or entirely. In my mind, an honest exploration at the point of contact is a valuable and rewarding process.

For example, when I first started working with adult sex offenders, I discovered countertransference unlike any I had experienced in the past. I became uncertain of my own ability (or willingness) to work with clients who had this particular problem, and I remember consulting with a colleague about the intensity of these feelings and the way they destabilized me. My colleague counseled me to make efforts to develop sensitivity to sex offenders—something I found challenging but not impossible. I began by listening to her as she described to me the personal histories of many of the sex offenders she had treated. As I listened, I heard stories reminiscent of those told by my clients who were adult survivors of abuse. It didn't take long to realize that we were sometimes discussing the same population. Many sex offenders have their own histories of severe abuse, and although there is no linear causal relationship between past and current behaviors, I came to view the two as connected: Histories of abuse contribute to maladaptive adult functioning, particularly repetition of dysfunctional patterns. As I understood this correlation, my sensitivity grew. It then became apparent to me that I could be sensitive to the history of abuse and its inherent pain, without excusing the behaviors that caused pain to others.

What I learned in this process is that it is important for us as therapists to be sensitive to each person's experience by trying to listen and understand without being defined and limited by our countertransference. When we work across cultures, countertransference abounds—based on a complex interaction among our own backgrounds and experiences (which limit or increase our sensitivity to one degree or another), our prior exposure to cross-cultural work, our comfort with our own discomfort, and the internal pressure we feel to be sensitive (which in and of itself can promote a sense of discomfort).

Developing and enhancing sensitivity entail personal focus and applied effort. Some people are naturally sensitive and seem to have an inherent ease about them as they interact with others. For others, being sensitive implies more work, and some are more willing to do this work than others.

Another example from my own professional life has been trying to teach people how to work with children. Some mental health professionals are not naturally comfortable with children, and yet they may be in jobs that require some interaction with them. Frustrated and anxious, they come to training sessions to learn how best to interact with or evaluate children, in order to be of help. Again, the first step is to slow down, observe, listen, and try to become sensitive to a child's experience of the world. Although this sounds simple, it can be challenging to shift from "doing something" to "being with" in an effort to connect, to touch and be touched emotionally, and to gain insight into the child's internal life experience. Establishing sensitivity allows the clinician to forge a relationship, which then in turn develops trust and creates a starting place for assistance.

Obtaining Knowledge Responsibly

The second level of response is to gain the knowledge and tools required in order to be of assistance. Doing this responsibly implies accountability for our insights and subsequent behavior. Mental health professionals have the responsibility to recognize their own limitations, practice within their area of knowledge, consult with or refer to others when limitations cause obstacles, and uphold the basic medical principle "First, do no harm." Most ethical guidelines emphasize these basic tenets because of the vulnerability of clients seeking assistance and the implied power differential when clients pay "authorities" to help them.

Becoming licensed to practice psychotherapy is a long, strenuous process of learning about self and the use of self in the best interest of others. However, acquiring a license (and the independence it bestows) does not imply an endpoint in the development of the therapist role. Instead, most mental health professionals are required to seek out continuing education in order to maintain the necessary knowledge and skills to be competent professionals. The trouble is that gaining knowledge alone does not automatically translate into responsible behavior. Obtaining knowledge and skills must be followed by practice and maturity.

Gaining knowledge is done in many ways: reading, attending lectures, watching videos, taking classes, and so forth. However, probably the most powerful way to learn is to "practice with accountability"—that is, to work in front of experienced colleagues. Allowing exposure and inviting commentary on one's work are humbling and powerful experiences that usually yield valuable feedback and direction. Each mental health professional will operate within a personal comfort zone in respect to learning, and with the advent of Internet courses that offer continuing education credits, it's possible to learn in the privacy and safety of one's own home. Nevertheless, I encourage mental health professionals to defy their own tendencies to avoid accountability, and to consider obtaining knowledge in a variety of traditional, nontraditional, and more exigent ways.

Developing Active Competence: Moving from Knowledge to Behavior

The third and last level of response is the development of active competence, which can only be attained after introspection leads to the building of sensitivity and awareness, which in turn elicits the desire to learn. Once knowledge and skills are obtained, the task is immense: The development of competence inherently means a change in behavior and the development of an action plan. Sadly, many stop short of translating their desires and skills into action, and my hope is to stimulate some thinking about how this response level is attained.

Here's the trickiest question of all: "How do I convert what I know into what I do?" This is an incredibly complex process that often seems impossible. For example, I can know on an intellectual level that children are intimidated by adults, that they are often hesitant to talk to adults, and that they may find coming to therapy intimidating and unfamiliar. That is, I may have the knowledge "Put the child at ease," or "Help decrease the child's anxiety," but how do I convey this knowledge through action? How do I know what to do, particularly if I feel my own internal pressure and anxiety to perform well? This question must be tackled generically and then applied to cross-cultural work (which may elicit even more anxiety).

The knowledge is available, and skills have been learned (and, ideally, practiced). Now the process follows a predictable path: An interactive, circular pattern of thought and response must take place. Attention must be paid to internal experience, the response to that experience, the behavioral attempt, and the reshaping of this attempt based on external feedback.

Here's an example: A therapist thinks, "Oh, this kid is painfully shy. He won't make eye contact with me. Maybe he doesn't like me. My best joke fell flat. He looks terrified." This is the therapist's internal thought. Now the therapist checks in on his own feeling state: "My hands are sweating. I feel uncomfortable and anxious. I knew I shouldn't have taken this case. I'm better with outgoing, hyperactive kids." Now the introspection is underway.

Next, the therapist tries to empathize with the child. "Wow, he must be feeling really uncomfortable, even scared . . . wow, his little hands are shaking . . . poor guy . . . I've got to help him relax." The therapist has developed sensitivity, and this leads him to want to help. Now the knowledge has to be accessed: "Okay, I am going to tell him that I'm a little nervous in new situations myself, and then I'm going to show him around. I remember Dr. Polland did that in the videotape."

Now the therapist takes action and says, "You know, I hate going new places for the first time. Sometimes I get a little worried when I don't know what's going to happen. Let me show you the playroom and what's in here. Just for you to know, this is a place where kids play some of the time and talk some of the time. You decide what you want to do."

Coincidentally, the therapist is now feeling more relaxed. Now the child begins to look around with more curiosity, as the therapist focuses away from him and on the toys he's showing the child. The therapist notices that the child's hands have stopped shaking, and takes a minute to acknowledge that the first obstacle has been removed.

This is the process of converting knowledge into action. The therapist will now remain aware of self, behavior, and the client's response to each clinical behavior. The therapist will then continue with those behaviors that elicit positive responses and will develop a unique pattern of interactions with this child, based on this interactive, circular pattern of thought and response.

AHNNA REVISITED

At the beginning of this chapter, I have described a Chinese child, Ahnna, who was adopted by a Midwestern couple, Scott and Joelle, after Ahnna's mother and grandmother both died and her father was unwilling to become her caretaker. Ahnna's father was grief-stricken when his young wife died in childbirth, and he seemed anxious to forget the past, remarry, and parent another child. Ahnna's gender reportedly also dissuaded him from meeting his parenting responsibility. Scott and Joelle had gone through rigorous fertility treatments and had been unable to conceive. They both came from large families and had eagerly agreed to have five children (a number that represented the average of both sets of siblings). They were profoundly distressed at their inability to conceive, yet embraced the concept of adoption with abandon, in spite of cautions from both sets of parents (Ahnna's reluctant but loving adoptive grandparents) about adopting a child who was not European American, who was not an infant, and whose history was unknown. Scott and Joelle felt bewildered when Ahnna developed a long list of problem behaviors—not only because they didn't know what to do to help their child, but because they felt they could not turn to their parents for help. By the time they came to treatment, they were stressed out, frustrated, and fraught with helplessness. I now provide highlights from the evaluation and treatment, particularly as it relates to cross-cultural issues.

Assessment

I met with Scott and Joelle to gather their psychosocial information and histories, which were unremarkable. Both came from intact families, had lots of siblings, had experienced the privilege of good educations, had enjoyed positive community life, and were not able to identify any serious stressors in their combined past (except for Joelle's loss of a neighbor/friend in a car accident). Their medical histories were benign, and both enjoyed good health, as did their extended families. There was no alcoholism, violence, or mental illness in their families, and they wanted nothing more but to provide a loving home for their daughter.

When I asked about their decision to adopt a Chinese child, they quickly answered that they were told there were lots of Chinese babies available, and that the wait would be relatively short. They noted that they had had a 3-year wait and were signed up with several agencies. "We just wanted a healthy baby. We didn't care where the baby came from, although China and Russia seemed to be countries where everyone said there were fewer problems getting a child."

I pressed a little more about their decision to adopt a Chinese child by asking what they thought about an interracial adoption—that is, what issues they had anticipated, given the merging of cultures. They looked at each other and had very little to say. Finally, Scott said, "Our focus was on getting a baby. We think she's beautiful, and the fact that she's Chinese is kind of irrelevant." Now it was my turn to be stunned. "How can a child's culture be irrelevant?" I asked myself, but at this point I responded, "The Chinese culture is full of rich traditions and quite fascinating. It might be interesting for you to learn a little about it, since Ahnna is Chinese." I said this in my most gentle voice, but Scott was a little perturbed with me: "We need help with the fact that she humps the furniture. Her being Chinese has nothing to do with that!" I backed off immediately. "I agree with you 100%. She's having a number of problem behaviors, and we have to find a way to help her with those behaviors first."

I then shifted the conversation to the standard gathering of information, such as when each problem behavior had begun, what Scott and Joelle had done that helped or made it worse, and whether there were times of the day or locations in which the behavior increased or decreased. Finally, I asked the parents to tell me about what was going well with Ahnna. Joelle immediately called Ahnna "a little angel, sweet and loving." Scott added, "She's a little pistol, very bright. She's speaking English really well, even though she didn't know a word when we first got her." "Wow," I said, "children are amazing. Imagine her being bilingual at her very young age." The parents looked puzzled: "Well, we're not sure how much Chinese she might speak. We couldn't understand her at first, and the agency said that she was really shy." "Sounds like she's grown out of her shyness, which is a good sign," I stated. Joelle and Scott became more relaxed as they were able to articulate positives about Ahnna. I reiterated and emphasized what I had learned from them: "Sounds like you both are very eager to be good parents, and you've got a beautiful little Chinese daughter, Ahnna, who is having some adjustment problems right now. These are probably temporary, but stressful nonetheless." Scott remarked, "You're the first person who's used the word 'temporary'; everyone else seems to be 'doom and gloom.'" When I inquired about his sources, both mentioned their parents.

Building Sensitivity

I have had a few other Chinese clients, but not more than 10 or so. I have worked with many interracial adoptions, but most of the children were from Central or South America; I've seen a handful of Russian children. My first-level response was building sensitivity through introspection. I imagined what it was like to grow up in the Midwest, live a simple family- and community-oriented life, fall in love in college, and be single-minded about having a large family. (Believe me, this was a stretch from my own personal experience.) I did a kind of guided-imagery exercise about Scott and Joelle and their journey into adoption, including the 3 years of waiting. As good-natured, decent people, they disregarded cross-cultural differences and chose to select a child of any race and ethnicity. Their wait produced such angst that they accepted the first available child and had few concerns about Ahnna's being Chinese. They were actually the opposite of racists: They saw no racial identity in Ahnna at all, and I remember thinking that my job would be to ignite their interest in Ahnna's racial identity in order to maximize her potential to become a healthy, well-grounded Chinese American child and adult.

I had a great deal of empathy for Joelle and Scott on many levels, and yet my attention turned to Ahnna's adoption journey as well. She was born to a dead mother, and she had spent her first 18 months with a loving but ill grandmother who had died likewise. Ahnna's father had turned his back on her, and yet I felt saddened by his loss, not only of Ahnna's mother but of Ahnna as well. In pain, he had chosen to recreate a family but to leave Ahnna far out of his life; indeed, he might never know that the child had come to be raised in the United States. Ahnna had then lived in an orphanage that was reportedly clean and efficient, but her care was provided by many caretakers, and it's unclear how she adjusted to the loss of her grandmother. The agency guaranteed that she had been well cared for, but there are no guarantees in such a situation, and no one would ever be sure what this child's 3 years in the orphanage had been like. Then she was swept up into the arms of a young and willing European American couple, and was brought across the ocean to a new life full of new smells, sights, food, and language. I wondered how much disparity she could identify, and how she felt in the arms of these eager yet nervous young parents, who spoke to her in English and were taller, thinner, and blonder than most of her caretakers probably were. I wondered what her first impressions of this new country had been, and I was taken back to my own first journey from South America to Washington, D.C., when I was 7 years old and thrust into second grade to learn English. I did, but not without a lot of withdrawal into my memories and avoiding tears as I longed for my grandmother's smile and the wonderful breakfast she cooked for me each morning. I became very sensitive to the experience of each person in this case as I reflected on how far they had traveled to arrive at my door, once again full of expectations and hope. Immediately I felt moved to my second level of response.

Obtaining Knowledge Responsibly

I decided to do some reading on Chinese and Chinese American families, as well as on interracial adoption (many of these books have been cited earlier in this chapter). I also called a Chinese American friend, a social worker with whom I had shared cases, and I took her to lunch. I wanted to hear about her experience of immigrating to the United States with her family when she was 5 or 6; I wanted to know about her family, her schooling, her Chinese American bicultural identity, and much more. Our lunch lasted 3 hours, and we chatted about many common and unique experiences. She reminded me about a book I had recommended to her, *The Spirit Catches You and You Fall Down* (Fadiman, 1997); I reread it, finding a deeper level of meaning this time around. I was truly inspired by what I read, as well as by my friend Joyce (formerly Chung). The sensitivity and knowledge were merging and commingling, evoking ideas, plans, and eventually my third-level response.

Developing Active Competence:
Moving from Knowledge to Behavior

My first meeting with Ahnna provoked a little anxiety for her, evident in her clinging to her mother as her mother carried her into my office. I saw Joelle's frustration at having to carry her daughter up the stairs, and I heard it in her voice as she kept telling Ahnna that she was too big to be carried.

Joelle's frustration and irritation were obvious, but she complied with Ahnna's request to carry her, even though Ahnna was practically choking her with a strong embrace around the neck.

I greeted Ahnna by shaking her hand and bowing my head. I made sporadic eye contact and used a tempered voice. I showed her around my office, so that she could see what she liked and what she wanted to do. I told her that she could say as much or as little as she wanted. She wanted no verbal communication in our first meeting. She asked to get down from her mother's arms as soon as she saw the toys in the play therapy office. She explored quietly and nodded when Joelle told her she'd be outside waiting. Ahnna seemed to make a very quick adjustment to her new environment; Joelle later told me that she was shocked when Ahnna did not run after her or start screaming.

After walking around the room, looking with curiosity, touching and picking up many things, and setting them back down again, Ahnna seemed to freeze in place when she found a sandbox filled with smooth white sand. She immediately put her hands in the box, needing little permission to proceed. I explained that she could put miniatures in the sand and create a "world." I added that she could use as few or as many miniatures as she liked, and that there was no wrong or right way to build a "world." She grabbed a set of little Chinese dragons and proceeded to make a number of shapes with them—straight lines, boxes, and finally small and large circles. Her final first "world" in the tray was a circle with the Chinese dragons, two masks, and lovely pale crystals (Figure 1.1). She literally held the sandbox in an embrace when I told her it was time to go. She ran into her mother's arms and didn't look at me again as I escorted them out.

The next time Ahnna came, she made a beeline to the sandbox and proceeded to take out the Chinese dragons, masks, and pale crystals. This time she surrounded one of the masks in red crystals and placed it diagonally across from the other mask. She then put green trees (later, stones) around the second mask and drew lines with her finger in the center of the tray, making a sign. I was intrigued by the sign, and went to the Internet to look up Chinese letters and symbols. I was interested to find that she had drawn the symbol for "mother" between the two masks. The dragons were placed in dyads around the tray (Figure 1.2).

This play with the masks, dragons, finger writing in the sand, and crystals of light and dark colors continued for four or more sessions. By then, Ahnna had learned to time herself within our 50 minutes, stopping 10 minutes ahead of time so that she could explore the rest of the room. I was fascinated as I observed Ahnna's extraordinary abilities to "tell time" without a timepiece, structure her time so that she could engross herself with the sandbox, and then leave time for exploring the room. I surmised that these abilities with time were by-products of being raised in an orphanage.

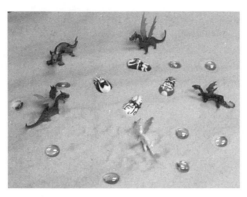

FIGURE 1.1. Ahnna's first "world."

The next toy to capture Ahnna's attention was a small Chinese doll in a crib. She seemed in disbelief when I told her that the doll had a high chair, a crib, a changing table, and a bathtub. I brought out the tub with warm water and soap. Ahnna looked cautiously around the room and then put her finger in the water ever so quickly, to make sure that I was giving her permission to bathe the baby. The bathing of the baby appeared disquieting, compelling, and almost sacred. She was in complete silence as she carefully undressed the doll, bathed her, and put on her pajamas. This doll came with Chinese clothes, and there were Western clothes in a bag as well. Ahnna used these clothes interchangeably, depending on what action she would take with the baby doll. When the baby slept, she put bright red Chinese pajamas on her. When Ahnna was going to feed the doll or take her to the park, she put Western clothes on her. By the end of treatment,

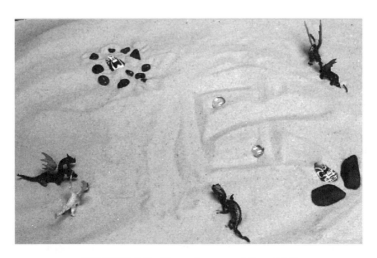

FIGURE 1.2. Ahnna's second "world."

Ahnna had altogether ceased dressing the baby doll in Chinese clothes; however, I had counseled Joelle to purchase some Chinese pajamas and dress wear for Ahnna, and she very much enjoyed wearing the pajamas to bed and dressier clothes to parties.

I met monthly with Scott and Joelle. Initially, I encouraged their patience, telling them that Ahnna was using therapy well and that her problem behaviors seemed clearly related to the transition she was making into a new country, a new culture, and a new family. They expressed some concern that Ahnna seemed to be "just playing" with me, and I gave them a little pamphlet to read about play therapy and explained once again that play therapy was serious work.

I put all of Ahnna's problem behaviors in the context of her making a normal adjustment. I commented that bedwetting and smearing feces were understandable signs of regression. The stress of the move had probably precipitated a temporary developmental regression in which she both reverted to earlier, less controlled behaviors, and at the same time elicited more primitive caretaking in her parents (a kind of reparenting). I informed them that according to recent research, masturbatory behavior in children is quite normal and seems to peak between the ages of 3 and 5. This caused Scott first to look bewildered and then to say gleefully, "Okay, so she's right on target with that behavior." I told them that it would not be uncommon for this child to masturbate as she drifted off to sleep to comfort herself, and that they should let me know if she began to masturbate in public. Joelle cringed when I said this, and I quickly reassured her that most children are quite responsive to distraction strategies such as putting something in their hands to play with (e.g., a ball or clay), as well as to encouragement to change location, do physical activity, and so forth. The parents seemed reassured. They also noted that Ahnna had had fewer altercations with children in school since coming to therapy (although this was probably just a coincidence).

I gave Scott and Joelle some other ideas about the difficulties experienced by Ahnna at this time. I told them that even though Ahnna had lost her biological mother in childbirth and had never actually known her, it was likely that on a subconscious level she was mourning the death of her mother (and mother country) and shifting her loyalty to her new adoptive mother.[1] I further advised them that they had a polite, creative, and smart daughter who was adjusting to a new life as a daughter to both a mother and a father (i.e., consistent caretakers of both genders), a new country, new routines, new food, new interactional styles among children, new pets, and novel eating and sleeping routines. She had endured tremendous challenges, and had found ways to elicit attention from others that were probably attempts to help herself with her fears, worries, and substantial losses.

As Ahnna developed a new expressive strategy in therapy—namely, "playing it out"—her behavioral problems decreased accordingly. In addition, Scott and Joelle quickly learned that their parenting strategies could help increase or decrease the problem behaviors. Their insights and willingness to follow advice and then generate their own creative interventions made working with this couple a delight.

I counseled Ahnna's parents about bedtime routines—in particular, not letting Ahnna drink fluids after dinner. I turned my attention to this behavioral strategy after referring them for a medical exam with a pediatrician to make sure that the bedwetting was not symptomatic of a physical problem. The doctor gave Ahnna a clean bill of health.

When I began working with Scott and Joelle about limit setting in general, and specifically about denying fluids after dinner, they were highly uncomfortable; they didn't like seeing Ahnna unhappy and, for the most part, gave her everything she requested. I told them I understood completely that they wanted to please and comfort Ahnna, but I emphasized that setting limits is as important to children's emotional development as nutrition is to physical growth. Slowly but surely, Ahnna found that her mother was setting a limit and sticking to it (as opposed to giving in once Ahnna complained), and she complied with drinking her juice at dinner and then going to the bathroom prior to bedtime. In an attempt to make the bedtime routine a little more fun, I encouraged the parents to think about a warm bath followed by bedtime stories. The parents told me that they gave Ahnna showers and not baths; their pediatrician had cautioned them against letting the child soak in bubbles because of possible urinary infections. I told Joelle that she could let Ahnna play in the tub (without bubbles) with some tub toys and wash her with soap once she was ready to get out. Ahnna loved this new routine prior to bed and seemed to go to bed relaxed.

I also suggested bedtime stories, and Joelle and Scott took turns reading to her. I was most interested in their reading books that might inform Ahnna about international adoptions and ethnic differences. I had learned through her play that Ahnna was quite aware of skin differences. As a matter of fact, when I asked her to make a self-portrait, she drew a very small girl with black hair and brown skin. She looked at all the brown pencils before finding (what she thought was) the perfect match. I remember her placing the pencil point against her arm to determine whether the shade was correct. When I asked Ahnna to draw a kinetic family portrait (a picture of "you and your family doing something together"), she colored in Scott's and Joelle's skin with a peach pencil (something Scott and Joelle found amazing, since they "never commented on differences in their skin color"). As I have noted earlier, it seemed that Scott and Joelle were color-blind to Ahnna's Chinese heritage—something I found well intentioned but misguided. I instructed them on the importance of discussing Ahnna's adoption, her birth country, and her unique skin tones, and eventually teaching Ahnna about the rich history and tradition of China. They were slightly reluctant at first, but they followed my advice and soon found themselves enthralled with a culture they had only seen as something incidental. It was their own idea to hire a Chinese tutor for Ahnna to make sure that Ahnna's Chinese was not forgotten. A side benefit was Ahnna's contact with a positive adult role model who could tell Ahnna about the "old country" as well as being in America. Scott and Joelle often consulted the tutor about important holidays and traditions. They had made a great shift and undertaken the goal of raising a bicultural child who might fully appreciate the contributions of both birth and adoptive backgrounds. Toward this end, I encouraged them to approach familiarizing Ahnna with her Midwestern roots as well. Scott brought home a map puzzle and instructed Ahnna about the United States of America. He also took a play airplane and would track both their own and Ahnna's journeys to the family they had created together.

Scott and Joelle kept in touch after therapy ended, giving me progress reports. Ahnna had become the apple of their eye, and they looked back with amazement at the acute difficulties they had experienced after Ahnna first arrived in the United States. They eventually moved back to their Midwestern hometown, and left the East Coast with a strong resolve to approach their families of origin with all the information they had acquired about China, true biculturalism, and acculturation.

SPECIFIC ISSUES IN CROSS-CULTURAL PLAY THERAPY

As noted in other chapters of this text, there has been a paucity of tangible guidance on cross-cultural play therapy. However, play therapists, like most other mental health professionals, need to recognize the significance of cross-cultural issues and to promote ongoing discussion of them. This book is intended as a springboard for additional introspection, dialogue, and proposed action.

Regarding play therapy specifically, there are obvious ways in which we can ensure that we maintain a competent cross-cultural focus when providing our services. Earlier in this chapter, I have discussed the three levels of response necessary to the development of cross-cultural competence in mental health professionals. Those three levels of response steer the establishment of a cross-cultural play therapy office. Therapists are urged to develop insight and sensitivity, which will lead to gaining knowledge, which in turn will lead to taking action.

Toys

Play therapists use toys to optimize and promote therapy goals. Every serious play therapist maintains an organized, categorized, purposeful list of toys that are age-, gender-, and culture-based. Toys are selected in controlled fashion in order to achieve different purposes; toys that elicit symbolic expression are most often utilized by play therapists. Toys that distract children, bring forth random or generic play, or overstimulate children are usually less in demand in play therapy offices. This is not to say that random or generic play isn't useful in and of itself, but it may be less valuable in the play therapy setting. There may also be very practical and desirable reasons for not distracting or overstimulating children.

In my experience, toys that spark symbolic communication and expression render the greatest benefits, and so I pay particular attention to selecting toys that can have ample applications. For example, a miniature representing fire has many broad symbolic uses: It can be used to suggest danger, excitement, sexuality, destruction, warmth, nurturing, or a force of nature. This is a much more useful miniature to have in a play therapy office than, for example, a cartoon character such as Nemo the fish or Spiderman. Although these figures are part of popular culture and children enjoy playing with them, the play they engender appears to center around the prepackaged stories of the characters. I don't mean to imply that some children won't boldly extract the characters from determined stories and endow them with completely original story lines, but this is the exception in therapy rather than the rule. The task, then, is to select carefully and unlock opportunities for exposure and expression.

Those who do sand therapy are already familiar with the use of miniatures. However, many play therapists are not trained in the use of sand therapy, find the process cumbersome, and shy away from utilizing so many props. Those familiar with sand therapy know that miniatures are categorized and kept in good order. The animal kingdom, for instance, can be categorized into prehistoric, wild, zoo, farm, and domestic animals. Sea creatures have a variety of subspecies that can be grouped together.

To continue with this sample category, cross-cultural play therapists pay attention to animals that are typical of other cultures and recognize the distinctive meanings afforded to animals in different cultures. In Japan, the snake is not a frightening creature; it's a symbol of wisdom. The owl, a symbol of wisdom in European culture, is viewed as a sign of death and dying among Native Americans. The iguana conjures up fear in many young children who don't live in tropical areas; however, iguanas are common play companions in Mexico. There are animals that are specifically associated with some cultures. For example, when people think of Australia, they think of kangaroos, koala bears, wallabies, and dingo dogs. China is known for panda bears, and Alaska and northern Canada are known for polar bears. My birth country of Ecuador is known for its giant turtles, aptly called "Galapagos turtles" for the area in which they live.

Other categories of miniatures merit equal thought. Structures, for example, are important to explore. China has pagodas, temples, and bamboo huts; different groups of Native Americans have tepees, sweat lodges, and longhouses. The list is endless, and it behooves us to make sure that our collections contain as many representations as possible of the world and its diverse and plentiful cultures. The greater the range of miniatures displayed in the play therapy office, the greater the likelihood that identification, projection, and processing can take place.

Play therapy offices should therefore contain as many visible representations of cultural diversity as possible. In addition to miniatures, special care must be taken in the selection of dolls, books, videos, and games in order to suggest diversity in language and in pictorial thought. More and more children's books are being written in different languages and depict children of varied skin colors. When musical instruments are provided, it is important to include a wide variety that nevertheless have universal appeal, such as drums, flutes, strings, maracas, and castanets. Certainly drums have enjoyed great popularity among many cultures and are still used in different combinations to create primary, distinctive cultural sounds. Canino and Spurlock (2000) encourage clinicians to establish an ambiance that reflects the cultural heritages of their various client populations. They discuss paying special attention to having additional dolls when working with children whose extended families are very involved in their lives; they also advise discussing favorite foods, birthday celebrations, heroes and heroines, and music, in an effort to understand a child's cultural context. Inclan and Herron (1998) decorate their clinic with maps and posters that will be familiar to their child clients. All these efforts send a consistent message to children: They are welcome; they are respected; and both their differences and their similarities are valued.

Therapist Behaviors and Actions

The personal behaviors of the therapist are also paramount to cross-cultural competence. Ahnna's case illustrates this point. Chinese people tend to emphasize formal demonstrations of respect among people. I knew that Ahnna would recognize a slight bow of the head as familiar, since she had lived in China for her formative years. It's possible that the slight movement of my head when I first met her allowed her to feel a little safer than she might have otherwise. Her mother told me that her staying alone with me so shortly after meeting me was quite rare for Ahnna.

Because of the respect that is maintained among people in China, I also sought to quiet myself when I met with Ahnna. I paid attention to my tone of voice, pattern of speech, and physical movement. I sat quietly as she played, and I conveyed calm and acceptance. I think this might have also had an impact on Ahnna's sense of security with a stranger.

As mentioned previously, I gained knowledge in Ahnna's case through reading and consulting with a colleague. I then applied the knowledge through specific actions, such as purchasing Chinese apparel for my Chinese doll, placing chopsticks along with the play forks and knives, reading books on biculturalism, encouraging Scott and Joelle to purchase traditional Chinese clothing for Ahnna, and having the parents tell and show Ahnna her immigration history (with a map and airplane). In addition, the parents hired a tutor so that Ahnna would not lose her first language, Chinese. They also promoted a relationship between Ahnna's tutor's family and their own, sharing meals and outings. Scott and Joelle read books about China and began to honor their child's biculturalism, rather than disregarding the rich traditions and values of Chinese culture. Both the parents and I discussed the process of acculturation with Ahnna directly, and the tone of her skin was no longer ignored, but celebrated.

Ahnna was helped to do some other important work in therapy as well. She represented her Chinese mother in her sand "worlds" and eventually said goodbye to her. Joelle and Scott participated in this ritual, designed to help Ahnna with her transition to her new family. Scott and Joelle read letters they had written to Ahnna's dead mother. In the letters, they thanked her for the gift of Ahnna's life. They told Ahnna's birth mother how they had hoped and prayed for a little daughter just like Ahnna, and how happy they were to welcome them into their lives. Then they told Ahnna's mother about their own upbringing and extended families and how they hoped to move back to the Midwest someday because they loved their birth state so dearly. Unexpectedly, they vowed that they would visit China with Ahnna one day, so that she too could see her place of birth. During this remarkable ritual, Ahnna used the little mask that she had included in her first and second "worlds," and that I hypothesized represented her birth mother. The family decided to give a burial to Ahnna's birth mother by planting a cherry tree in their back yard and burying the little mask next to the tree. They told me in my last conversation with them that they were taking the cherry tree with them on their Midwestern move.

SUMMARY

Play therapists have abundant opportunities to develop and implement cross-cultural competence in their work. I dare say that play therapists are better positioned than many other clinicians are to make visible and concrete efforts to honor diversity and acquire cross-cultural competence.

Becoming cross-culturally competent requires commitment and follow-through. No single action is sufficient, and there is no rigid endpoint. We must develop and then expand our insights, sensitivity, knowledge, and action language. A complex circular method of personal introspection followed by information gathering leads to skill building, action planning, and implementation. We must sustain this process rigorously with each child and family we meet. A broader definition of culture intimates that mental health professionals are constantly working cross-culturally, even though ethnic differences are most likely to elicit thought or discussion about cross-cultural work.

The emphasis on cross-cultural sensitivity has been actively upheld in the mental health profession for decades. Initial efforts were launched to raise awareness by providing education about diverse cultural groups. These data were valuable and provided the necessary context in which to identify problem areas and articulate needed change. Additional work by mental health professionals on task forces or committees of professional organizations advocated cross-cultural education for mental health professionals. Ethical guidelines were written that encouraged clinicians to evaluate themselves, explore their own cultural background, recognize biases, and make conscious efforts to deal with problem areas in order to provide responsible cross-cultural therapy.

Perhaps the area least explored has been the translation of knowledge into action. For instance, several licensing boards require that applicants seeking mental health licenses complete a course in cross-cultural competence. Astonishingly, however, some mental health professionals can complete such a course and remain completely unresponsive to and unmoved by the knowledge gained. They may feel the material does not apply to them or their clients; they may believe they are already functioning well enough; or they simply may be unwilling to make additional efforts to change their awareness, insights, or behaviors.

Those invested in becoming cross-culturally competent and responsible must practice the principles laid out in this chapter: building sensitivity, obtaining knowledge responsibly, and translating knowledge into action. The third response is the most challenging and requires the most forethought and follow-through.

As Athena Drewes and I have noted in the Preface to this book, we play therapists may be in a position to make the most facile transitions from knowledge to action, because play is a universal medium, toys are used routinely, and there is less import placed on verbal communication. As play therapists, we are much more likely to linger in the spheres of creative imagination, storytelling, fantasy, laughter, and play. We are also keen to access symbolic language, to use metaphor, and to externalize inner worlds. We are therefore more likely to be able to expand the lens through which we see (and understand) children's broad cultural worlds.

NOTE

1. I had seen hints of this in Ahnna's second sand "world," in which there were two masks, one juxtapositioned diagonally across from the other. The mask with the ring of red crystals may have been the mother she had lost, and the other mask, nestled among trees and later stones, gave the suggestion of life and nurturance.

REFERENCES

Allen, L. R., & Majidi-Ahi, S. (1998). In J. T. Gibbs, L. N. Huang, & Associates, *Children of color: Psychological interventions with culturally diverse youth* (pp. 143–170). San Francisco: Jossey-Bass.

Boyd-Franklin, N. (1989). *Black families in therapy: A multisystems approach*. New York: Guilford Press.

Canino, I. A., & Spurlock, J. (2000). *Culturally diverse children and adolescents: Assessment, diagnosis, and treatment* (2nd ed.). New York: Guilford Press.

Carter, R. T. (1995). *The influence of race and racial identity in psychotherapy*. New York: Wiley.

Fadiman, A. (1997). *The spirit catches you and you fall down: A Hmong child, her American doctors, and the collision of two cultures*. New York: Farrar, Straus & Giroux.

Falicov, C. J. (1998). *Latino families in therapy: A guide to multicultural practice*. New York: Guilford Press.

Gibbs, J. T., Huang, L. N., & Associates. (1998). *Children of color: Psychological interventions with culturally diverse youth*. San Francisco: Jossey-Bass.

Giordano, J., & Giordano, M. A. (1995). Ethnic dimensions in family therapy. In R. Mikesell, D. Lusterman, & S. McDaniel (Eds.), *Integrating family therapy* (pp. 347–356). Washington, DC: American Psychological Association.

Gopaul-McNicol, S. (1993). *Working with West Indian families*. New York: Guilford Press.

Inclan, J., & Herron, D. G. (1998). Puerto Rican adolescents. In J. T. Gibbs, L. N. Huang, & Associates, *Children of color: Psychological interventions with culturally diverse youth* (pp. 240–263). San Francisco: Jossey-Bass.

Koss-Chioino, J. D., & Vargas, L. A. (Eds.). (1999). *Working with Latino youth: Culture, development, and context*. San Francisco: Jossey-Bass.

LaFromboise, T. D., & Graff Low, K. (1998). American Indian children and adolescents. In J. T. Gibbs, L. N. Huang, & Associates, *Children of color: Psychological interventions with culturally diverse youth* (pp. 112–142). San Francisco: Jossey-Bass.

Lee, C. C. (Ed.). (1997). *Multicultural issues in counseling: New approaches to diversity* (2nd ed.). Alexandria, VA: American Counseling Association.

Lee, W. M. L. (1999). *An introduction to multicultural counseling*. Philadelphia: Accelerated Development.

Lu, Y. E., Lum, D., & Chen, S. (2001). Cultural competency and achieving styles in clinical social work: A conceptual and empirical exploration. *Journal of Ethnic and Cultural Diversity in Social Work, 9*(3/4), 1–32.

Mason, B., & Sawyerr, A. (2002). (Eds.). *Exploring the unsaid: Creativity, risks and dilemmas in working cross-culturally*. London: Karnac Books.

McAdoo, H. P. (Ed.). (1993). *Family ethnicity*. Newbury Park, CA: Sage.

McGoldrick, M. (Ed.). (1998). *Re-visioning family therapy: Race, culture, and gender in clinical practice*. New York: Guilford Press.

Paniagua, F. A. (1994). *Assessing and treating culturally diverse clients: A practical guide*. Thousand Oaks, CA: Sage.

Pinderhughes, E. (1989). *Understanding race, ethnicity, and power*. New York: Free Press.

Ramirez, O. (1998). Mexican American children and adolescents, In J. T. Gibbs, L. N. Huang, & Associates, *Children of color: Psychological interventions with culturally diverse youth* (pp. 215–239). San Francisco: Jossey-Bass.

Roysircar, G., Sandhu, D. S., & Bibbins, V. E. (Eds.). (2003). *Multicultural competencies: A guidebook of practices*. Alexandria, VA: Association for Multicultural Counseling and Development.

Sue, S., & Morishima, J. (1982). *The mental health of Asian Americans*. San Francisco: Jossey-Bass.

Tatum, B. D. (1997). *"Why are all the black kids sitting together in the cafeteria?" and other conversations about race*. San Francisco: Jossey-Bass.

Tseng, W.-S., & Hsu, J. (1991). *Culture and family: Problems and therapy*. Binghamton, NY: Haworth Press.

Uba, L. (1994). *Asian Americans: Personality patterns, identity, and mental health*. New York: Guilford Press.

Webb, N. B. (Ed.). (2001). *Culturally diverse parent–child and family relationships: A guide for social workers and other practitioners*. New York: Columbia University Press.

Zimmerman, T. S. (Ed.). (1991). *Integrating gender and culture in family therapy training*. Binghamton, NY: Haworth Press.

2

Play in Selected Cultures

Diversity and Universality

ATHENA A. DREWES

> Play, a dominant activity in all cultures, is viewed to be a cause and an
> effect of culture. Play is an expression of a particular culture; play is an
> important context or vehicle for cultural learning/transmission, as well
> as an indicator and reflection of child development. (Roopnarine &
> Johnson, 1994, p. 5)

Play is a universal, natural, and pleasurable experience, and for children
it is an integral part of their lives. Play's very nature is social and the social
is inextricably linked to culture (Brown, Sutterby, Therrell, & Thornton,
2000). While play is universal, the way play looks and works differs across
and within cultures (Sutton-Smith, 1974, 1999). Throughout history, play
has had a very significant impact on the development and continuation of
culture (Monroe, 1995). It is through play that a society is able to express
its view of life and its place in the world; play is how it develops poetry,
philosophy, music, dance, competition, and social structures (Huizinga,
1949). It is through such play-based activities as children's games, dance,
music, storytelling, family tradition, and festivals and celebrations that
culturally based behaviors are introduced and passed on from generation to generation (Monroe, 1995). Play can affect a culture's development
through giving children opportunities to explore and interact with objects
and individuals; to master their own bodies and surroundings; to build
relationships; and to practice and organize both new and old skills (Allison,
1992; Barnett, 1990; Kelly & Godbey, 1992; Monroe, 1995). Through these

opportunities, the survival of individuals increases—allowing for the successful integration of such behaviors into social structures, and thus in turn for cultural survival (Monroe, 1995). Play is also important in the development of values—a system of beliefs, ethics, and actions that guide each individual. Through play, children learn about their society's rules and acceptable behaviors (Monroe, 1995). Finally, children learn to sort out what is and is not like them, and what these differences mean in their culture as compared to other cultures (Levin, 2000). Children learn through play who is an appropriate play partner, who can play what roles, and the meanings that play has. Society socializes the child depending on their environment and play is part of how children are socialized through learning cultural activities and games that are passed down through generations (Sutton-Smith, 1999).

Societies learn gambling, risk taking, survival skills, community, independence, and rules of engagement with others, which defines the personality of the society (Brown et al., 2000). Play deprivation has serious consequences as nonplayers are ostracized from group activities and thus it is the social characteristics of play that are the key element to how we learn to get along with one another (Frost & Jacobs, 1996).

Although play is believed to be universal, the amount of attention devoted to play in a particular society depends in large part on the cultural beliefs about the nature of childhood, and on the specific goals by caregivers for their young children (Vandermaas-Peeler, 2002). Play can be considered one of the most vital activities for children in all cultures (Bloch & Pellegrini, 1989). It serves many important functions for children's development, including cognitive skills (e.g., symbolism and language use, problem solving, role play, and creativity) and forming social relationships (e.g., friendships, social competence, emotional maturity) (Vandermaas-Peeler, 2002).

Play is seen in many cultures as an essential feature or characteristic of childhood—as a way to understand the very meaning of human existence (Oke, Khattar, Pant, & Saraswathi, 1999). So important is play that most societies have made provisions for it (Sutton-Smith, 1986). Cultural norms and opportunities determine how different kinds of play are stimulated, and whether adults see play as a good thing or a waste of children's time. They also determine whether the adults encourage work versus play, whether children have freedom for exploration and motivation to practice adult roles through play, and whether the environment provides easy access to materials and models for creative and constructive play (Edwards, 2000). Culture and tradition are critical in determining how much and in what ways children are allowed and encouraged to undertake such imaginative and cognitively enhancing play. Play with toys, for example, is hypothesized to be "mediated through social interactions and social traditions" (Sutton-Smith, 1997, p. 8). Children all over the world engage in various forms of play, be it with dolls, balls, homemade materials, or through their own imagination and creativity (Vandermaas-Peeler, 2002). Hughes (1999) calls play a "true cultural universal." Regardless of the child or family's economic situation, children seem to find both time and materials for play. In fact, Schwartzman (1986) argues that children play even more creatively when ready-made toys and their own private space are not available.

Recently, researchers (e.g., Farver, 1999; Farver & Shin, 1997; Gaskins, 1996; Haight & Miller, 1992, 1993; Roopnarine, Johnson, & Hooper, 1994) have begun to explore the cultural dimensions of children's play and a body of research on sociocultural variations of play has been developing. Sociocultural variations of play depend not only on the attitudes of parents, teachers, and society in general, but also on such variables as the amount of play space and time available to children (Roopnarine, Lasker, Sacks, & Stores, 1998). Recent sociocultural research suggests that pretend play has a role in meaning making in human cultures (e.g., Farver, 1999; Gaskins, 1996; Goldman, 1998; Haight, Wang, Fung, Williams, & Mintz, 1999; Lancy, 1996). Both theorists and researchers concur on a common set of characteristics that distinguish play behaviors from nonplay behaviors for children across all ages, domains, and cultures. Isenberg and Quisenberry (2003) identify these unique features, which include behaviors that are (1) intrinsically motivated and self-initiated, (2) process-oriented, (3) nonliteral and pleasurable, (4) exploratory and active, and (5) rule-governed. As a *process* play facilitates individual understanding of skills, concepts, and dispositions; as a *product*, play provides the vehicle for children to demonstrate their understanding of skills, concepts, and dispositions (Fromberg, 1998, 2002).

A culturally sensitive theory of development, one that seeks to understand how a child and culture are cocreated, has begun to emerge (Haight et al., 1999). While play is often assumed to be universal in its characteristics, researchers and theorists are challenged to understand play as a culturally mediated activity that may take different forms in different groups.

Play is also significant for the development of young children themselves. The United Nations' "Declaration of the Rights of the Child," and the United Nations Educational, Scientific, and Cultural Organization's International Children's Charter, accord play equal importance with nutrition, housing, health care, and education (Kim, 2002). Through play, children learn how things work; find out how to solve problems; talk and share ideas with others; develop and express imagination and creativity; learn about themselves, others, and the world; and discover how to express feelings in a healthy way (Spodek & Saracho, 1988). Erik Erikson (1963) has argued that childhood play is a metaphor for adult life, and that play allows children to become partners with their future, along with parents (Bruce, 1993). Play can be a measure of a child's social, emotional, cognitive, physical, and language development (Eisert & Lamorey, 1996; Eisner, 1990; Smilansky, 1990). Margaret Donaldson (1978) has stated that children need to make sense and derive meaning from the context of their lives. Through play, indeed, they can create their own context. Catherine Garvey (1977) believes that play's giving children this kind of control is the most important contribution it makes to their development. Play can also provide children with the sense of power that comes from being able to master new and different experiences, as well as ideas; this results in feelings of accomplishment and confidence in themselves as they learn to work out new concepts and experiences (Levin, 2000).

Sociocultural theories have emerged to help understand play and pretend play in children. Piagetian theory predicts that children's early pretend play will be similar across diverse cultural groups (Haight & Black, 2001). Anthropological reports suggest dramatic cross-cultural variation in pretend play. In the past 17 years researchers influenced by cultural psychology, activity/practice theory, and other sociocultural approaches have begun to articulate a culturally sensitive theory of play, which seeks to understand how universal and culturally variable aspects of play interact in specific communities, which in turn creates distinctive developmental pathways for play (Haight & Black, 2001). Comparative research points to a number of potentially universal characteristics of pretend play (Haight & Black, 2001).

Piaget (1951) described play as a medium for children's intellectual development and for the formation of flexible thought and creativity. Consistent with Piagetian theory, children begin pretend play at about 12 months of age in communities in which children are seen as unique and where priority is given to supporting development and individual achievement. Adults in such cultures see pretend play as a way of facilitating children's development and creativity, and adults in turn offer active support and elaborate and encourage pretend play (Haight & Black, 2001). In communities where adult work is seen as a priority, children also begin pretend play at about 12 months of age. No particular developmental significance is given to pretend play by the adults, and children are not actively encouraged to pretend (Gaskins, 1999).

Russian theorist Lev Vygotsky (1967, 1990) saw play as the leading source of development in preschool years, and emphasized its importance for both cognitive and affective development. Vygotsky proposed that play was one of the most important sources of learning for young children, and that learning occurs primarily through observations and interactions with highly skilled members of the culture (Vandermaas-Peeler, 2002). Indeed, playing with a more sophisticated partner such as an adult or an older child will enhance the child's skills and encourage more complex play (Howes & Unger, 1989). In order to help the child develop more advanced skills and to reach the end goal of independence, parents and others provide enough help and support so the child will not fail at the task, yet not so much that the child will not be challenged (referred to as *scaffolding*) (Vandermaas-Peeler, 2002). Creative, innovative, and imaginative play requires prowess, competence, craftsmanship, and skills that children acquire during life (Bruce, 1993); these are universal aspects across cultures. Play with toys, for instance, is vital for enhancing and fostering symbolic knowledge "in the individual mind . . . to stimulate the child mind to further growth and development" (Sutton-Smith, 1997, p. 7).

There is a rapidly growing body of evidence that play is not only central but critical to childhood development (Frost, 1997). For a variety of species, including humans, play can be nearly as important as food and sleep. It is indeed serious business (Frost, 1997). Sutton-Smith (1997) has concluded that play has multiple motivations and functions for child and human development. Repetitive physical play in infancy is seen as improving children's motor skills, whereas exercise play in childhood increases strength and endurance, and rough-and-tumble play serves to develop fighting skills and controlled dominance, especially in males (Pellegrini & Smith, 1998).

In the Western world in particular, the phenomenon of play has become of interest to researchers over the past several decades, as the value of play for young children has been recognized (Sutton-Smith, 1985). The research has confirmed many of the points made above. For instance, not only has play been found to lead to discovery, reasoning, manipulative skills, divergent thinking, and improvement in problem solving, but all sorts of learning—about information, about people, and about customs— are embedded in play (Yeatman & Reifel, 1992). Through play, children practice many of the skills they will need as adults (Frost, 1997). The first-hand experience of play involves struggling, exploring, discovering, practicing, and problem solving (Bruce, 1993). The intense sensory and physical stimulation that comes with playing helps to form the brain's circuits and prevent loss of neurons (Begley, 1996). Play also provides opportunities to learn social roles and rules, as well as a socially shared system of symbols, including language (Yeatman & Reifel, 1992). Through adult support, play can provide an effective way to work on various concepts and skills, from understanding and celebrating diversity to practicing basic literacy and numerical skills (Levin, 2000).

Bronfenbrenner (1979) offers an ecological model that emphasizes the various systems embedded within a culture that influences how a culture regards or values play. Each society may have definitive views about whether children should be protected from adult work or be part of it, whether or not they should have a "protected social space to play" (Garbarino, 1989) and how play fits into a child's development within the "macrosystem" in the midst of various social systems, with the family occupying a central role (Bronfenbrenner, 1979).

Based on their study of children's play in six cultures, Beatrice and John Whiting (1975) concluded that children in more complex cultures play more and with more complexity. Within the most complex groups, there was more play in children who had greater freedom to roam about the community and play with whomever they chose (Sutton-Smith & Roberts, 1981). The critical variable in the amount of parental support for the role of play hinged on the need to involve them in the economic survival of the family. In societies where children must work to help support the family from an early age, there is less observation of play than in societies where children are less tied to the economic well-being of the family (Vandermaas-Peeler, 2002).

The nature of parent–child interactions during play differs widely by culture and socialization. Adult beliefs about play influence how likely parents become involved in their children's play and even those beliefs can differ widely by culture. And while parental support of play is extremely important, the actual means of support—be it through providing space, materials, or social interaction—can also vary widely by culture. For example, when mothers did not consider themselves appropriate play partners for their children, East Indian, Guatemalan (Goncu & Mosier, 1991), Mayan (Gaskins, 1996), and Mexican mothers (Farver, 1993) were much less involved and engaged in the play than American and Turkish mothers, who in turn saw play as culturally appropriate behavior (Farver & Wimbarti, 1995; Haight, Park, & Black, 1997). In many cultures, it is the older siblings who guide and are responsible for the younger children's play. Farver (1993) found that in Mexican families, older siblings offered guidance to and involved their younger siblings in complex pretend play, which was similar to that of American mothers with their young children. This was in contrast to sibling play in the United States, which was more conflictual (Farver, 1993). In contrast, in Mexico older siblings are more likely to be play partners with their younger siblings, and there is a much more nurturing relationship between older and younger siblings.

Similarly, Farver and Wimbarti (1995) found Indonesian parents responsive to their young infants' needs until they are mobile, at which point the older siblings take a more active role and the parents no longer are play partners with their children. In addition, the study found that children's object play and cooperative social pretend play followed trends similar to those of Western children. Older children offered encouragement of younger children's play, whereas Indonesian mothers used more directives and corrections of their children's behavior (Vandermaas-Peeler, 2002).

When adults do engage in their child's play, how they interact varies in part due to socialization values and goals. Haight and colleagues (1999) found European American mothers emphasized independence and self-expression, while Chinese caregivers were more interested in social harmony and respect for rules. They also found that Chinese children had more social play and the initiation of Chinese caregivers' play was often focused on practicing proper conduct. In contrast, they found that Irish-American children had longer periods of pretend play by themselves, alternating with social pretending with peers. Japanese mothers tended to focus more on social interactions and communication in play with their young children, while American mothers tended to use play for teaching world knowledge (Tamis-LeMonda, Bornstein, Cyphers, Toda, & Ogino, 1992). Furthermore, American mothers who were primary caregivers were highly engaged in their young children's pretend play, but as the children grew older pretend play became a joint activity (Haight & Miller, 1993) and mothers incorporated their children's pretending into daily routines of laundry and cooking. Haight and Miller (1993) also found that mothers were their child's primary play partner until age 36 months, and that their child preferred this arrangement to their older siblings. After age 3, mothers arranged more play dates with friends and were less likely to play with them.

Another universal aspect of early pretend play is that it is essentially social in nature (Haight & Black, 2001). Naturalistic observations in the homes of European American (Haight & Miller, 1992), English (Dunn & Dale, 1984), Turkish (Goncu & Mosier, 1991), Mexican (Farver, 1993), and Chinese (Haight et al., 1999) families show that pretend play develops primarily in interactions with others. In Taipei and Chicago, naturalistic observations reveal considerable variability in social functioning, content, and conduct of the caregivers in pretend play (Haight et al., 1999) with Chinese mothers teaching Confucian principles to their children through their concern for proper conduct during adult–child interactions as a rehearsal for formal interactions with a teacher. European American mothers were much more child-centered and supported their children's individuality and self-expression. They initiated only half of the interactions and followed their children's lead, supporting and elaborating on their children's ideas. However, one must be cautious in assuming similarities across cultures have the same underlying belief system (Haight & Black, 2001). For example, African American and Chinese caretakers appeared to similarly emphasize impeccable conduct while pretending with their children. But when examining this further, Haight (1999) found that Chinese mothers supported such impeccable conduct as an index of virtue, but African American mothers supported it as a survival skill in a hostile environment. Furthermore, the pretend play of young European American children revolves around realistic toys, while a significant proportion of Chinese children's pretend play involves no objects at all. American children use the shared scripts suggested by their toys to initiate social play, whereas Chinese children appear to use their shared knowledge of social routines to further their joint play (Haight et al., 1999). Therefore, the study of play or the interpretation of it should always be conducted with the particular cultural context in mind.

In some cultures, competition in play can be a motivating and stimulating force that can spur individuals toward greatness. The skills and values needed for survival are perpetuated through games and sports. Game playing further leads to growth in self-esteem and self-worth, self-discipline, and dependence, as well as the development of skills in working cooperatively (Bunker, 1991; Schroeder, 1995). Indeed, games can reflect many aspects of culture, as the values, interests, and activities of the specific groups who play the games are studied. Anthropologists studying ancient peoples discover that each group played games unique to its time, place, and environment (Barta & Schaelling, 1998). The rules for these games were invented, then ritualized over time, and modeled some aspect of reality (such as trading, hunting, warring, or strategic planning). Play materials came from the natural surroundings and environment. Games helped to build community, allowed for practice of skills, challenged intellect, and improved problem solving while simultaneously being fun (Barta & Schaelling, 1998). Studies of children's games across Britain (Opie & Opie, 1988) have found that once children understand the rules of games, they can become creative, break the rules, change them, or make up their own.

As integral vehicles of play, toys have a substantial impact on children and on themes in play. Toys and their value have been defined differently from culture to culture and over time (Kim, 2002). The use of play materials facilitates children's play activities by allowing for self-initiation and imagination, as well as interaction with parents, other adults, or peers (Kim, 2002). Spontaneous pretend play of European American, middle-class children typically occurs in relation to objects, notably toy miniatures such as dolls, cars, dishes, or telephones (Haight & Miller, 1993). But in cultural groups where such items are scarce (Heath, 1983) or are nonexistent (Gaskins, 1996), children enjoy active play using material at hand (Roopnarine, Hossain, Gill, & Brophy, 1994). Parental perceptions of what is a useful toy and for which gender, and how much to join in or not with a child's play, varies from culture to culture. Ethnicity and socioeconomic status (SES) may also influence the way in which preschoolers communicate and use toys during social interaction (Quay & Pinkett, 1986). Parents in some industrialized societies give children specific toys to promote certain skills and cognitive understanding, instead of fun (Kim, 2002). In addition, cross-cultural studies have shown that whether or not parents are involved in their children's play has a significant impact on language, cognitive development, and the ability to engage in symbolic and imaginative play (Bradley, 1986; Gottfried, 1986; Moore, 1968; Ware & Garber, 1972). Furthermore, creative and imaginative play is seen as more relevant and evident in open than in closed societies, as more valuable to foragers than to tillers, and as differently expressed in boys versus girls. It was most common in complex societies where children are allowed exposure to new and different things, or have more freedom to roam about away from their homes and to choose their playmates and companions (Edwards, 2000).

Children enact culturally specific themes reflecting activities and values important within specific communities. For example, children in the Marquesas Islands pretend to paddle canoes, hunt, and fish (Martini, 1994). Children in India enact traditional celebrations and folktales (Roopnarine et al., 1994). Korean American children focus on family role themes, while European American children focus on fantasy themes such as superhero adventures (Farver & Shin, 1997). In Chinese families where space was limited and children had relatively few personal possessions, they typically did not construct props from other available materials. Rather, a sizable proportion of their pretend play involved no objects at all throughout the age range and they relied on shared knowledge of social routines to keep expanding their play (Haight et al., 1999).

It is hoped that this chapter will help readers in their professional work as play therapists to become more culturally sensitive and competent. Ramirez (1988) wrote that by the year 2000, 40% of all public school students would be from ethnically diverse families (i.e., families whose backgrounds are not mainstream European American). Indeed, in at least 25 of the nation's largest cities, at least one-half of the students are from linguistically and ethnically diverse groups (Rettig, 2002). It is estimated that there are more than 106 different ethnic groups in the United States (Rettig, 2002), with 25% of U.S. citizens belonging to one of the four major ethnic minority groups (Glover, 1999). In 1996, the U.S. Bureau of the Census predicted that nearly 10 million Asians would move to the United States between the years 1990 and 2010; it was projected that the Asian population would be 12,121,000 in the year 2000 and 17,188,000 in the year 2010 (Lee & Childress, 1999). There are an estimated 30,587,000 Hispanics in the United States, about 11% of the total population. Mexican Americans represent 64.3% of the total U.S. Hispanic population—a young, diverse, and quickly changing population that is experiencing rapid growth (U.S. Bureau of the Census, 1998). Other U.S. Hispanic groups include Puerto Ricans (10.6% of the total), Cubans (4.7%), and Central and South Americans (13.4%). The proportion of the white non-Hispanic U.S. population by 2050 is expected to be just over 50% (Glover, 1999). As the number of culturally diverse individuals in the United States increases, we play therapists need to better understand both the diversity and the universality of play across cultures.

This chapter explores the various components of play in a selection of cultures, including cultural differences in parent–child play interaction and the use of games and toys. The emphasis is on ethnic differences, but other types of cultural differences (SES, etc.) are also considered, as are the features of play shared by almost all cultures. Through this material, it is hoped that readers will obtain a better understanding of the types of cultural issues that influence both parents' and children's view of play. In turn, readers will then be better able to advocate for opportunities and ample time for sustained play to occur, along with supplying the necessary materials that represent the diverse experience of the children we come in contact with. As play therapists, we need to be culturally sensitive to the fact that some children need time to play alone, in pairs, or in a group. Children from different cultures also require different amounts of time to demonstrate technical prowess, control, and mastery, as well as to understand the ideas, feelings, and relationships that play evokes (Bruce, 1993). Finally, we need to realize that no one can be expected to know everything about every culture. However, we can learn something about the most common patterns within the populations we commonly serve, while keeping in mind the fact that there is tremendous variation both within each group and among individuals. The best advice I can give readers is this: Don't be afraid to ask people about their culture, and share with them information about your own!

The following studies offer the reader some guidelines in how various cultural groups may view play, play materials, and interaction with their children. However, caution should be used in assuming that these studies are generalizable across the entire cultural group, as there is much diversity and differences within each.

PLAY IN EUROPEAN AMERICAN CULTURE

Parent–Child Interaction

Middle-SES European American mothers are reported to favor authoritative parenting with an emphasis on independence; they regulate interactions with their children in order to foster physical and verbal individuality and assertiveness in the children, as well as interest in the external environment (Bellah, Madsen, Sullivan, Swindler, & Tipton, 1985). The culture stresses values that foster individual achievement, self-actualization, and autonomy in children, and it heavily favors innate ability (Bornstein, 1994).

European American fathers have been found to spend more time with, and to play more actively with, their sons than their daughters (Bunker,

1991). Themes of caregiver–child pretend play reflect socialization values and goals, with European American caregivers generally emphasizing individuality, independence, and self-expression (Haight, Wang, Fung, Williams, & Mintz, 1999). Narratives within European American families often highlight children's positive and unique characteristics.

Toys, Games, and Types of Play

European American mothers tend to facilitate children to use toys functionally (Kim, 2002). Parents often choose specific toys for their children because the toys will elicit various types of roles. Sex-typed toys are often purchased, with one study of children's rooms (Rhinegold & Cook, 1975) finding a great difference in toy arrangement or preference. Boys' rooms were filled with toy animals, vehicles, military toys, and spaceships; girls' rooms had dolls and dollhouses, kitchen stoves, and tea sets. In another study, favored fantasy games of boys included adventure themes, fantasy characters, superheroes, and television-inspired roles, while girls showed a preference for family roles (Goldstein, 1994). However, similar patterns of toy preferences have been reported among children of European and Asian descent (Kim, 2002).

"Orchard Town" in New England, a small, low-income, predominantly European American town of 5,000, was part of a six-culture study (Edwards, 2000). The 24 children studied (aged 3–10) were found to score the lowest in responsible work, and the highest in access to toys, manufactured games, and store-bought play materials, of any group of children in this research. Girls scored higher than boys in playing games with rules. These youngsters lived in small families with few adults and children, and spent many hours indoors. Their parents encouraged them to entertain themselves by playing alone or together, with adults sometimes joining in, answering questions, or mediating disputes as needed. Role plays included having a birthday party, cooking, making beds, shopping with money, and dressing and taking care of baby dolls. Fantasy play was imaginative and included playing sheriff and deputies, riding horses (using objects to represent the horse), telephone calling, riding a "magic carpet" (a tiny rug), and using marbles to represent people. Creative/constructive play included follow-the-dot games, coloring, cutouts, drawing, building with blocks, cutting up magazines, sculpting with clay, and playing with a dollhouse. Books and television also occupied the children's time, along with board and card games.

Even where there are physical space constraints, European American caregivers still purchase large quantities of toys for their children (Haight & Miller, 1993). In games, urban European American children tend to be more competitive and less cooperative than rural children and children from other and mixed American cultures (Avellar & Kagan, 1976; Kagan, 1978). The European American culture encourages independence, competitiveness, and self-reliance, often in sharp contrast to other, more group-centered cultures (Cook & Chi, 1984).

PLAY IN AFRICAN CULTURES

Kenya

Edwards (2000) found that Kenyan children were absorbed into the work of their mothers, helping with agricultural work, animal care, and child care. They were discouraged from leaving their homesteads, in order to minimize aggression with neighbors. Children played with their relatives in mixed-age groups and often combined play with their work, which was not hard labor. In taking care of the infants and toddlers, the older children would use imitation, laughter, playful touching, and teasing in interactions. The boys would play in ways that could be interrupted while they were herding cattle and goats in the pastures. The games were not competitive ones with rules, but rather tag and dirt-throwing contests. Toys were few and mostly simple, homemade ones such as slingshots (Edwards, 2000).

Liberia

Lancy (1977) noted over 90 forms of play in Liberia, which were grouped into eight major categories: (1) *Nee-pele*, make-believe; (2) *Sua-Kpe-pele*, hunting play; (3) *Pele-Seng*, toys; (4) *Pele-Kee*, games; (5) *Polo*, storytelling; (6) *Mana-Pele*, dancing; (7) musical instruments; and (8) *Kpa-Kolo-pele*, adult play. Children would play out dramatizations of real-life activities, such as imitating the work of a blacksmith. Hunting play also involved make-believe imitation of actual situations, with rules and turns taken. The variety of games was quite large, and many games exhibited a developmental progression in complexity (Lancy, 1977). For example, *Tiang-kai-sii* was a simple counting game with 10–25 stones, played by children aged 8–11. The complexity of the game increased for children aged 12–15, and it was then called *Kpa-keleng-je*. There were relatively few traditional toys, mostly dolls for girls and tops for boys. The children would convert natural materials and objects into toys. In storytelling, animals talked to each other and to people; humans had access to magical powers; and there were spirits in human form (e.g., witches). Stories were told from the age of 9 upward (Lancy, 1977). The board game *wari* or *mancala* was also played, taught to teenagers by their grandfathers or other kinsmen who were greatly senior to them. There did not seem to be games that involved throwing or batting balls, only kicking balls (Lancy, 1977).

Much of the imitative play was a prerequisite for actual adult work and served as an apprenticeship of sorts for the children. With the influx of Western development, the Western games and variations of play began to be incorporated within the culture as well.

Zambia

Zambia lies in the high interior region of southern Africa; its people primarily speak Bantu and traditionally live by a combination of cattle raising and agriculture. Leacock (1976) found that as children took on adult roles during imitative play, they were praised and applauded. For instance, the children would learn by observation and play being chief with elders and a court; they conducted mock proceedings and gave "judgments" with heavy penalties. The most commonly observed physical play was soccer, with many teams and endless variations of the game. In addition, games such as hide-and-seek, tag, hopscotch, tug-o-war, and jump rope were played. Boys and girls characteristically had their own types of games and would play separately. A common girls' game involved throwing a ball back and forth between two lines of players, trying to hit a girl in the center before she could fill a bottle with dirt. Playing the "husband and wife" game (Leacock, 1976) entailed building and making thatch houses and clay utensils. Both sexes made clay cattle and other objects, with the girls often making dolls and household utensils, and the boys making tools and cars. "The most characteristic of African toys is the wire car that most boys start making at eight or nine and are one to two feet long, and made of heavy wires bent into shape and bound together with finer ones" (Leacock, 1976, p. 471).

Hunting games were also not unusual, with the children setting fire to dry grass in the fields to catch rats, and making slingshots to shoot birds and trap them with *ulibo* (a plant gum that they collected, heated with oil, and kneaded). Natural materials and items in the environment were used to make musical instruments, with children writing their own songs and organizing bands. Girls would dance *chitelele* (a traditional woman's dance), stepping out of a singing, clapping circle to dance individually in the center. Folktales were also told by the older children to the younger ones. Other games played by the children included variations on marbles and jacks played with stones, as well as board games of various sorts—including checkers (the favorite) and *nsoro* (similar to *mancala*, using a board with carved-out hollows into which pebbles were placed for playing).

PLAY IN AFRICAN AMERICAN CULTURE

Parent–Child Interaction

Ericksen, Yancey, and Ericksen (1979) observed that middle-SES African American fathers were more involved in household tasks and child care than are middle-SES European American fathers. Low-SES African American mothers were found to play more frequently with their infants than middle-SES mothers of infants did, whereas children in the middle SES initiated play more often and did so verbally more frequently than their low-SES counterparts (Hammer & Weiss, 1999).

Socioeconomic level as well as the safety or lack of safety of the community in which the child lives also impact the quality of the child's play. African American families are 10 times more likely than European American families to live in neighborhoods where at least 30% of the residents are poor (Duncan, Brooks-Gunn, & Klebanov, 1994). African American families are also disproportionately represented in neighborhoods characterized by high violence, crime, and drug activity (Sampson, Raudenbush, & Earls, 1997).

Letiecq and Koblinsky (2003) reported on a study of 61 African American Headstart fathers and father figures in violent neighborhoods. They found that the male caregivers were most likely to adopt the strategy of monitoring and teaching personal safety, followed by teaching neighborhood survival tactics, reducing exposure to violent media, engaging in community activism, and instructing children to fight back. The male caregivers would permit their preschooler to play on playgrounds only when directly supervised by an adult, and kept them from playing video games that contained a lot of violence. While such close supervision and confinement may be critical to keeping children physically safe, such restriction may hinder young children's ability to explore their environment, cultivate social relationships, master motor learning skills, and achieve other developmental milestones (Holland, Koblinsky, & Anderson, 1995). Restricting children's neighborhood contact, literally keeping children out of sight of one's friends and neighbors for safety reasons, runs counter to African American values of child-centeredness (Hill, 1993). Several fathers in the study noted that there were no longer grandparents and other surrogate parents on the street to nurture, teach, and discipline their children. Although some fathers attempted to counterbalance neighborhood dangers by taking their young children to safer environments (e.g., parks, malls, recreation centers in nearby suburbs), such strategies do not build the social support networks that formerly characterized their inner-city neighborhoods (Letiecq & Koblinsky, 2003).

Other studies (e.g., Jarrett, Jefferson, & Roach, 2000; Mohr, Fantuzzo, & Abdul-Kabir, 2001) have shown African American mothers keeping their children close and providing constant supervision/chaperoning, teaching practical household safety skills (e.g., not sitting by windows) and restricting neighborhood activities (e.g., use of community playgrounds).

Toys, Games, and Types of Play

Black Americans have nurtured and created a dynamic culture within a climate of intense racial, social, and economic exploitation and injustice. Kinship networks, religious beliefs, and families infused with their values and cultural knowledge have developed (Saloy, 1999). Black Americans have maintained a lively and widespread verbal art tradition in both urban and rural communities, forming a separate culture within the dominant culture, which remains predominantly oral (Saloy, 1999). In New Orleans, stories, song, and other kinds of black folklore continue to develop. Oral lore includes many traditional forms such as children's sidewalk and jump-rope rhymes, handclap songs, and rap, as well as toasts and tales recited by adults, each representing a unique cultural response to a difficult historical and economic climate (Saloy, 1999). African Americans have long had storytelling as an important component, with singing or chanting of long oral narratives concerning gods, heroes, and demons (Saloy, 1999). In New Orleans, the verbal artistry among African American children is expressive and creative and contains a necessary developmental function. Sidewalk songs pass on attitudes and knowledge about the self, imitations of adult life, and values and distinct criticisms of adult life and society's norms (Saloy, 1999). Children's folklore is play but it is also a comment on the world with some of the attitudes imposed by race, sex, family, ethnic, and economic influence. The children learn the oral songs and rhymes of sidewalk games from other children, but also from their parents even before they learn how to speak. The existence of children's sidewalk culture comes from the adult culture, which believes that children should socialize separately, not be part of adult talk and play with other children. Sidewalk songs take the place of nursery rhymes and it fulfills the function of reflecting and criticizing society while transmitting values. The child is not only entertained by the folklore but it also teaches them how to manipulate words, develop their group identity, learn about gender roles, create a bond, teach them how to handle verbal or physical abuse (being able to "rap" or "jive" oneself out of a fight or punishment), and provide an opportunity to practice interacting with authority (Saloy, 1999). But perhaps the most important cultural component is that when the children perform the sidewalk songs they practice and learn to contribute to the rich African American verbal culture (Saloy, 1999).

Play is also utilized as part of religious and cultural rituals. Kwanzaa is a cultural celebration in December that has seven principles based on

African harvest rituals. Kwanzaa was established in 1966 by Dr. Maulana "Ron" Karenga, a scholar and social activist. It was created in order to help African Americans remember their heritage (Cady, 1996). During Kwanzaa children are taught a rock-passing game, "Oboo Asi Me Nsa Nana." The children sit in a circle and sing while passing the rock counterclockwise, which reinforces the third principle of cooperation (Ujima) in Kwanzaa. The children tap the rock on the ground and pass it to the next person in rhythm to the beat of the music. If a child breaks the rhythm, they are out of the game. It is a game of precision, accuracy, rhythm, and cooperation (Cady, 1996).

Qualitative differences in the sociodramatic play of economically disadvantaged African American preschool children were noted by Weinberger and Starkey (1994). There were less diversity and variation in roles used in play, less advanced object utilization, fewer verbalizations during play, and fewer numbers of participants in sociodramatic play. Girls spent more time in sociodramatic play than boys did. Functional play episodes occurred most often and were the longest in duration as compared to constructive play and pretend play. Other researchers have found that low-SES African American children are less socially interactive with their peers during pretend play (Udwin & Shmukler, 1981).

PLAY IN ASIAN CULTURES

Within the United States, many people tend to stereotype Asians, or to assume automatically that all Asians or Asian Americans are either Chinese or Japanese. However, there are over 40 different Asian groups living in the United States, and thus Asian Americans cannot be viewed as a homogeneous entity (Stevenson, Stigler, & Lucker, 1985). There is much diversity among Asian groups and cultures. Lee and Childress (1999) define the geographic differences as follows:

1. *Pacific Islanders:* People from Hawaii, Samoa, Guam, and other small Pacific islands.
2. *Southeast Asians:* People from Vietnam, Thailand, Cambodia, Laos, Myanmar (formerly Burma), Singapore, Malaysia, Indonesia, and the Philippines.
3. *East Asians:* People from China, Japan, and Korea.
4. *South Asians:* People from India, Pakistan, and Sri Lanka.

Although there are four distinct groups listed, there are many subgroups within each group, which often differ in terms of language, religion, customs, history, and race (Feng, 1994). Again, the temptation to view

Eastern (or Western) cultures as monolithic and homogeneous, rather than as multifaceted and pluralistic, must be avoided. This section addresses only those Asian cultures encountered through a review of the literature, and therefore it is not an exhaustive account of all the Asian cultures listed above. (Indeed, the intent throughout this chapter is to look briefly at only a selection of cultures, rather than to provide an exhaustive discussion.)

Bali

Storey (1977) found that children in the small village of Piliatan, on the Indonesian island of Bali, were often engaged in the working world of sweeping, raking, shoveling, planting, and carrying rice and water on their heads. Little play occurred as they carried out these responsibilities. The children, even those under 5 years of age, were responsible for caring for the babies. Children's leisure activities often consisted of sitting, staring aimlessly into space, eating, and talking quietly. However, they would play with kites, pinwheels of bamboo, and flowers, and would engage in such physical activities as hopping, jump rope, climbing trees, turning somersaults, and playing with animals. Storey also noted 28 games, many of which were similar to European American games. The majority emphasized physical skill, such as trying to hit another running child with a stone, chasing, and tag. Four were games involving strategy in finding a hidden item based on the opponents' facial expressions. Another four games were based on a mythical story theme, but these were not the games of preference for the children; this fact perhaps reflected acculturation to the influx of tourists, which created a desire for money and material possessions (Storey, 1977).

Although children in Bali are "casteless until puberty," the status they achieve in their games "prepares them for positions they are to assume in the adult social order" (Storey, 1977, p. 80). Imitative play reflected adult activities; it increased during times of festivity, when the children would imitate temple festivals and performances. These festivals and performances were family events lasting all day, which allowed not only for entertainment and relaxation in a social group, but also the acquisition, appreciation, and sustaining of the Balinese culture. Children would imitate cockfights (which they were not permitted to watch, but often peeked at), as well as cremation, which was another temple festival event. "This was a huge, joyful sendoff of the soul to higher and better worlds, and with the potential for reincarnation. The body was placed in an animal-shaped coffin and put into a huge colorful tower, which was twirled around to confuse the bad spirits, and then on fire to burn in magnificent splendor as everyone shouted with pleasure" (Storey, 1977, p. 81). The cremations were costly, and their preparation demanded much time and effort in making elaborate decorations. Much of the children's time was spent watching these preparations and attending the ceremonies, with some of the children imitating the events. Much imitation of the dancers performing the Ketjak Dance (Monkey Dance) was also noted. Fantasy play was not observed, which seemed in accordance with other cultures that were rigid, strict, highly stratified, and strictly regulated (Storey, 1977).

China

Parent–Child Interaction

Middle-SES Chinese mothers living in compact single-family apartments in Taiwan generally viewed pretend play as helping to facilitate development in their young children. They engaged in a higher proportion of such play with their children than middle-SES European American mothers did (Haight et al., 1999). The Chinese mothers' interactions were described as heavily didactic during pretend play, compared with those of Euorpean American mothers. They were directive and demanding of mature behavior, expecting the children to listen attentively to their elders, understand what was said, and behave accordingly. The Chinese mothers would also extensively show their children models of proper conduct, often focusing on those values and behaviors necessary for group acceptance and participation (Haight et al., 1999). Pretend play was often used to help teach such conduct: "Confucian thought has emphasized 'playing rites' in which children enact roles to learn social rules and adult customs" (Haight et al., 1999, p. 1479). Other investigators have found that personal storytelling is used to convey moral and social standards (Miller, Wiley, Fung, & Liang, 1997). Chinese caregivers generally emphasize harmonious social interaction obtained through obeying, respecting, and submitting to elders; adherence to rules; and cooperation (Chow, 1994; Pan, 1994). Narratives within Chinese families focus on moral and social standards (Haight et al., 1999).

Haight and colleagues (1999) found that Chinese children pretended more with their caregivers, whereas Irish American children pretended more with other children. In addition, Chinese caregivers initiated a relatively greater proportion of interaction with their young children than did European American caregivers, who tended to respond more frequently to child-initiated play. Other research has noted that Chinese culture stresses kinship, obedience, luck, fate, chance, and cooperativeness (Hsu, 1961), with life situations to be determined by circumstance outside one's control. Consequently, Chinese and Chinese American boys will exhibit more cooperative behavior than European American boys (Cook & Chi, 1984).

Toys, Games, and Types of Play

The Chinese children studied by Haight and colleagues (1999) had a modest number of possessions relative to European American children, although their mothers spoke of them as "spoiled" with respect to material possessions. The children owned collections of toy miniatures, stuffed animals, and a few toy cars or a doll. In the Chinese families, where space was limited and children had relatively few personal possessions, children typically did not construct props from other available materials. A sizable amount of their pretend play involved no objects at all throughout the age range studied. The children appeared to rely upon shared knowledge of social routines to propel their joint play and fantasy (Haight et al., 1999), not upon objects.

India

Parent–Child Interaction

The play profile of middle- and lower-SES children in India was studied by Oke and colleagues (1999). The urban cities of Mumbai and Vadodara in western India were used for the study. Adults, if present, would take one of three distinct roles in the children's play: They were either (1) instructive, telling the children what to do; (2) restrictive, cautioning and protecting them from something harmful; or (3) participative, playing with the children. The most frequently observed role was restrictive.

Toys, Games, and Types of Play

Play has considerable historical significance in India, with the presence of traditional toys and artifacts having been found in the Indus valley at Harappa and Mohenjodaro and dating back to 2500–1700 B.C. (Oke et al., 1999). These toys were indigenously prepared from naturally available materials like sticks, clay, and leaves. Some current toys, like the "snake toy," have ritualistic associations; others, like the "jumping monkey" or "acrobat," are for amusement. Play in Indian culture has been viewed as a "microcosm of an experimental theatre, wherein children learn adult rules and norms of behavior appropriate to the cultural context" (Oke et al., 1999, p. 209). The urbanization of India has resulted in a high-density population living in high-rise buildings, with consequent slum and ghetto settlements, restricted open spaces, and high levels of pollution. As of 1992, an estimated 75 million children under the age of 15 years lived in India (Bose, 1992).

The children studied by Oke and colleagues (1999), regardless of space, material, or other children to play with, had play as an integral part of their daily life. The more disadvantaged children in particular converted almost anything they could find into play materials or a play activity. Among middle-SES children, play was influenced by the presence of play equipment, such as swings, slides, and jungle gyms, along with the presence of adults. Play locations were much more limited for low-SES children, who often played in the street barefooted or used limited open spaces with heavy traffic, overflowing garbage, and people using the outdoors for washing clothes and dishes. Play materials among these urban poor children included rubbish lying around, plastic bags, bottles, wooden pans, empty tins, scraps of paper, and the like, which were creatively made into toys or games.

Some of the play reflected the traditional games played worldwide, like tag, hide-and-seek, and ball-and-stick-games, while other activities were modifications of those games. The modifications were often the result of restrictions posed by the environment. Pretend play included being film stars and using dialogues from films. Festival rituals like Ganapati (in honor of the elephant-headed god Ganesh) and Navratri (invocation of the goddess Durga for nine nights) were played, with children singing the fast beat of cinema songs to contrast with the lyrical traditional songs (Oke et al., 1999). As much as 75% of the play involved physical movement—chasing, jumping over obstacles like a wall or puddle of water, racing, and dancing despite limited space. Sedentary play included singing songs, rhyming games, making mud/sand pies, or rearranging twigs or stones in the environment. It was also not unusual to see a girl holding a sibling on her hip and playing at a public park, or young rag pickers chasing one another in play while picking rags. Even while helping their mothers wash dishes or clothes, children would play with the water and splash their feet and hands. "The child snatches an opportunity to play whenever possible" (Oke et al., 1999, p. 212).

By contrast, Edwards (2000) observed that in Khalapur, a farming and herding community of low SES, the children had a lot of leisure time but little play time. At home they engaged in much idle interaction, standing about, because the courtyards were crowded and they were discouraged from playing. Mothers often interacted in a scolding and reprimanding way and did not seem to encourage play.

Types of Group Interactions. Oke and colleagues (1999) noted that group games usually followed a specific pattern. The first step was the starting of a game, with children choosing and defining roles, and trying to get the best role using a method of chance. This might involve a jingle, a rhyme, or motor skills (e.g., each child would place a foot in a marked circle, and whoever removed a foot last was "it"). Next came marking boundaries and defining the limits of behavior for each player. In "teacher–teacher," the person playing the teacher could not smile! Then came the actual playing of the game, with lots of high-pitched voices and concentrated moves and strategies. The final step involved the dissolution of the game, which usually resulted from conflict among the players, from time running out, or from external interference (Oke et al., 1999).

Children played in the company of other children, when not alone, and preferred to play in homogeneous age and gender (see below) groups, but would play with whoever was available. Other than in the school setting, children rarely got a chance to play with single-age peers. Usually multiage groups played together, with the younger, inexperienced players assigned an insignificant role; this allowed them to learn the game through observation, like apprentices (Oke et al. 1999).

Gender Differences. Oke and colleagues (1999) found that girls and boys preferred to play in segregated-gender groups, which also was reflected in the types of games played. Girls preferred hopscotch or "four corners," playing with dolls, singing, and dancing. Boys preferred playing cricket, *kho-kho*, ball games, and cops and robbers. Girls would make out the boundaries first before initiating play, or would use corners in a classroom or space near the teacher's desk. Boys created the boundaries as a game proceeded, and usually chose open spaces. Girls tended to conform to the games' rules and to enforce them as well, while boys used flexible rules and conveniently changed them (Oke et al., 1999).

Edwards (2000) found that in Khalapur, the boys had much more freedom to roam, with the older ones watching after the younger ones (who were not expected to take care of cattle before the age of 6). The boys played games in the pasture, such as jacks and forms of hockey. They had few toys, but often played with sticks or bits of paper or cloth, being creative in using natural materials to construct their own toys. The girls also would join in using natural materials for making things to play with, but would also spend time alone embroidering, often without maternal assistance except for criticism of the work when shown (Edwards, 2000).

Japan

Expression of Feelings

A comparison of Japanese and U.S. preschool children's responses to scripts and symbolic play of conflict and distress (Zahn-Waxler, Friedman, Cole, Mizuta, & Hiruma, 1996) found significant cultural differences. The U.S. children showed more anger, aggressive behavior and language, and under-regulation of emotion than did the Japanese children. Japanese children were less likely than U.S. children to acknowledge negative emotion in a forced-choice situation. In the context of interpersonal conflict, U.S. children had a broader range of positive as well as negative behaviors than Japanese children. The U.S. children were much more ready to use force and aggressive solutions to solve problems than were the Japanese children; this appears consistent with the reported lower rates of violence and antisocial activity in Japan (Zahn-Waxler et al., 1996).

Relative to adolescents from Western cultures, Japanese adolescents show less aggression on projective measures, and more guilt and shame (Kornadt, Hayashi, Tachibana, Trommsdorff, & Yamauchi, 1992).

Expressivity is valued by Japanese mothers, but not as much as by U.S. mothers (Zahn-Waxler et al., 1996).

Parent–Child Interaction

An early study found that Japanese mothers emphasized soothing behaviors, whereas U.S. mothers engaged in more activities related to stimulation and exploration (Caudill & Weinstein, 1969). In another study, Japanese mothers were seen as offering greater promotion of interdependence than U.S. mothers, who promoted independence in their children (Weisz, Rothbaum, & Blackburn, 1984). Discipline practices tend to encourage Japanese children to learn what others feel (Lebra, 1976), whereas Western mothers are more accepting of aggression and sometimes less responsive than Japanese mothers (Kornadt et al., 1992).

Japanese children appear to have strongly internalized sanctions regarding issues of bringing harm to others (Zahn-Waxler et al., 1996). This is of note, given that in Japanese culture young children's negative behaviors, such as tantrums and being demanding, are viewed as age-appropriate during preschool years and are often more readily tolerated and even indulged (Tobin, Wu, & Davidson, 1989) than in Western culture. Anger and aggression, however, are incompatible with the broader cultural goals, including efforts to live in harmony with others. Thus these values may lead Japanese mothers to discourage harm doing in their children, as it may threaten the existence of an interdependent self (Zahn-Waxler et al., 1996). Furthermore, Japanese mothers more often use reasoning, strong negative emotions, disappointment, and guilt induction, in order to focus their children's attention more on the consequences received from others for hurting them.

Japanese mothers were noted to encourage their children to participate in interpersonal interactions in make-believe play, in contrast to U.S. mothers, who encouraged their children to use toys functionally (Tamis-LeMonda, Bornstein, Cyphers, Toda, & Ogino, 1992).

The cross-cultural differences noted here may be of long-standing origin, including centuries of differences in religious and political traditions in Eastern and Western cultures. "Confucian teachings stress control of emotions and impulses. Buddhist influence emphasizes nonaggression, acceptance of inhibition, quietness and (from a Western perspective) over-controlled behaviors" (Zahn-Waxler et al., 1996, p. 2474). Governmental systems have a further impact, through differing emphases on the rights of individuals in the context of the larger social order.

Taira, Okinawa

In a comparative study of six cultures, 24 children (aged 3–10) from a small village of 700 people relying on subsistence agriculture were studied in Okinawa (Edwards, 2000). The villagers spoke Hokan and Japanese. The children were found to have the highest play scores of any group in the study. The mothers and fathers were heavily involved in physical work, but the children had much freedom to wander and play in the open, welcoming courtyards. Children younger than 5 were seldom given chores, and they attended a community nursery school in the morning. The teachers taught turn taking and other skills that facilitated playing games with rules. The older children supervised the younger ones after school, with all playing in large groups. The children were resourceful in using many of the natural materials nearby for creative/constructive play. They would draw figures and house plans in the sand, make mud-pie trucks, write with chalk on the wall, dig gravel pits, and make houses of bamboo sticks. Their fantasy play included acting out a sword fight, playing house, telephone calling, using blocks and bits of wood for vehicle games, and playing ghost. Role play included playing house, playing store, and animal care. For group games, they chose marbles, wrestling, shooting rubber bands, and chasing one another (Edwards, 2000). Role playing dropped off at the age when children were required to begin playing a significant role in the household.

Korea

Parent–Child Interaction

In a comparison study of Korean and European American mothers of 1-year-olds, significant cultural differences were noted (Hupp, Lam, & Jaeger, 1992). The parents of the European American children more often selected rocking a child who was crying for no apparent reason than did the parents of the Korean children, who offered food instead. Parents of the European American children more often selected or provided play materials to a child who was demanding attention while the parent was busy, in contrast to giving the child something to eat or drink, which again was common for the Korean parents. Korean mothers' general tendency to use food as a strategy for comforting their children has been attributed to cultural child-rearing practices, whereby continuous and immediate gratification is given. Children are breast-fed whenever they cry, because it is presumed that they are hungry (Han & Washington, 1988).

The parents of the Korean children were more likely to select punishment in response to a child's doing something wrong (in contrast to stopping the child from doing the behavior) than were the parents of the European American children. And the parents of the Korean children more often elected putting breakable items away (rather than teaching the child not to break things) than did the parents of the European American children.

Hupp and colleagues (1992) also found that Korean parents intervened significantly more during the play sessions than did the European American parents. They perceived that their children had more of a desire for more adult guidance, and less of a wish to be independent, than the European American parents perceived. Child-rearing attitudes differed around various strategies used for responding to children's attention-getting efforts and managing their behavior. Hupp and colleagues noted that Asian mothers have high expectations for their children's success and believe that play is an important role in promoting this success. These authors further noted that "in the Asian culture, independent exploration by an individual is not valued as highly as it is in the Western culture" (p. 129). They attributed these findings to the Korean culture's deep influence by Confucianism, which values interdependence rather than independence and where the individual is conceptualized as a relational being. They also attributed their results to another deep-seated Korean child-rearing belief (Han & Washington, 1988) that infants should be well protected, since they are considered "to be physically and mentally unstable, sensitive and fragile beings, at risk from excessive external sensory or psychological stimuli" (Hupp et al., 1992, p. 129). Consequently, such general exploration as mouthing objects or toys by infants could be regarded by Korean mothers as risky behavior.

In a study of 409 Korean mothers of 3- to 5-year-olds in Seoul (Kim, 2002), the mothers were found to play more with their children than the fathers did. Mothers played with their children using toys for 36.7 minutes per day during weekdays and for 42.2 minutes per day during weekends, whereas the fathers played on the average only 15.1 minutes with their children during weekdays and 40.5 minutes a day during weekends. The longer a child played with toys, the longer both parents played with the child using toys.

Toys, Games, and Types of Play

The Korean parents assessed by Kim (2002) believed that toys were effective to facilitate children's interest in play and pleasure (36.1%), to improve children's creativity (31.5%), to develop positive feelings (10.3%), to promote physical development (9.2%), or to enhance intellectual development (6.7%). These mothers more rarely thought that toys were essential for facilitating language development and for acquiring Korean culture. Kim also found that the most common toy items that parents purchased included children's books, miniature cars or other small vehicles, writing or art materials, robots that could be assembled and manipulated by children, puzzles or pegboards, and electronic toys. Gender differences were noted, with boys receiving more cars, other vehicles, and war toys, whereas girls received more computer games, house sets, puzzles, and pegboards. The children who chose the more traditionally sex-preferred toys were more likely to have traditional mothers. A total of 45.2% of the mothers would choose imported toys for their children, ranking durability, safety, better designs and colors, age-appropriateness, and educational effectiveness in order of preference. Two out of three parents encouraged their children to go together with them to buy toys. However, after purchasing toys, parents spent little time playing with their children; two out of three children played with the toys either alone or with their siblings (Kim, 2002).

Some of the most popular games played by Korean children are *Gong-Khee Norhee*, *Ba Ram Gae Bee Norhee*, *Jae-Ghee Norhee*, and *Paeng-I Norhee* (Lee & Childress, 1999).

1. *Gong-Khee Norhee* (Jackstone or Pebble). The game can be played by oneself or with no more than six people. Five small stones each are needed to play. It is like playing jacks. The player needs to pick up one jackstone very carefully without touching the others, to toss the jackstone into the air, to catch it, and also to pick up the other jackstones from the floor (number determined in advance) one at a time before the tossed stone falls. The game has variations of throwing all five jackstones and trying to catch them all at once in the palm of one's hand, or with the palm facing downward (more points are earned for this). Those children not playing, or those who have lost their turn for failing to reach the final stage, chant a spell at the other players or make a funny face to have the others make a mistake and lose a turn. Benefits to this game include development of observation and concentration, problem-solving practice, intellectual development, and practice in adding numbers.

2. *Ba Ram Gae Bee Norhee* (Pinwheel Game). This game is played with at least one player and up to any number. Each player makes a pinwheel out of colored paper and a wooden stick. The children run around to watch the pinwheels spin. Benefits include gross motor development, entertainment, the pleasure of feeling wind, and the use of inexpensive materials.

3. *Jae-Ghee Norhee* (Shuttlecock). One to any number of players are needed. Anyone can play at any age, but it is usually considered a boy's

game. Coins or bottle caps and colored vinyl shopping bags are used to construct shuttlecocks. The goal is to keep a shuttlecock floating in the air, using only the feet (no hands). After kicking it into the air, players must stomp a foot before kicking it again. Players can use both legs to kick, kick the shuttlecock into their mouths so they can drop it again to kick, or kick it as high up over their heads as possible. Whoever kicks the highest wins. Benefits include physical and balance development.

4. *Paeng-I Norhee* (Toy Top Game). One to any number of players are needed. The game is traditionally played by boys, mostly in the winter, and can be played on ice. It requires two toy tops and whipcords (2-foot-long sticks with cotton strings attached to one end). Each player throws a top on the ground by unwinding the whipcord hard and fast, and tries to make the top hit another one; and the top still spinning after the collision wins. Benefits include practice in eye–hand coordination, development of concentration and observation, and physical development.

The Philippines

Parent–Child Interaction

In the study of six cultures mentioned earlier, Edwards (2000) studied 24 children (aged 3–10) in Tarong, a small hamlet of only 269 people in Luzon, the Philippines. The people only spoke Iloco and had a subsistence agriculture economy. The mothers were busy, but used work to keep their children occupied, along with organized group games. Adults were almost always nearby and were able to oversee their children.

Toys, Games, and Types of Play

Older children went to school, but afterwards would supervise the younger ones, taking great care to teach them how to play a variety of games with rules. These included hide-and-seek, tag, drop the handkerchief, junior versions of school games, and fantastic versions of baseball or basketball that bore no resemblance to the originals (Edwards, 2000).

Boys role-played smoking, planting and harvesting, cooking and eating, ironing, pounding rice, and having sex. Fantasy play included playing ghost, jeep, train, horse, and sword fight; make-believe bicycle riding; pretend card playing (using leaves); and performing pretend music. In creative/constructive play, children utilized natural and found materials to make mud pies, toy cars of cups and cans, guns out of bamboo, houses of branches, and whistles out of banana stalks. The study noted long periods of harmonious and constructive, cooperative play (Edwards, 2000).

PLAY IN HISPANIC CULTURES

As noted earlier in this chapter, there is much diversity among Hispanic groups, as well as within each group.

Argentina

Bornstein, Haynes, Pascual, Painter, and Galperin (1999) found that Argentine child-rearing values tended to stress obedience, reward, and punishment, with mothers promoting interactions intended to foster mutual dependence within the mother–child dyads. Middle-SES mothers tended to blame themselves for failures of child rearing, with self-descriptions indicating that they were reflective, self-critical, and fearful of committing child-rearing mistakes. Bornstein and colleagues also found that Argentine mothers tended to engage in more symbolic play as well as more social play with their toddlers, and to express more verbal praise toward them, than did U.S. mothers.

The play session and toys in Bornstein and colleagues' (1999) research served predominantly to mediate the interaction between Argentine mothers and children, as compared to U.S. dyads, for whom the play session was the stage and the toys were typically the objects of communication. Argentine mothers encouraged interactive, other-directed pretend play (e.g., feeding a doll or putting the doll to sleep), as compared to U.S. mothers, who encouraged functional play and combinations (e.g., dialing the telephone or nesting barrels). The Argentine mothers also displayed more positive affect than the U.S. mothers (Bornstein et al., 1999).

Mexican American Culture

Some research studies (Durrett, O'Bryant, & Pennebacker, 1975; LeVine & Bartz, 1979) concluded that permissiveness characterizes Mexican American parenting. According to other studies, however, traditional values and authoritarian structures are more characteristic of Mexican American child rearing (Kagan & Ender, 1975; Kearns, 1970). Such conflicting views indicate rather a broad range of parent–child interactions within this heterogeneous group. Anecdotal and nonempirical descriptions by Mexican Americans characterize child rearing within families as "warm, nurturing, and affectionate within a patriarchal, authoritarian family structure with its traditional extraordinary respect for males and the elderly" (Martinez, 1988, p. 275). Martinez (1988) found that mothers encouraged initiative in their children by limiting directives, along with frequently praising their children and knowing when to physically guide the children through solution of a task. Mothers who taught their children primarily through modeling failed to maintain their children's attention to the task. And children were more verbally negative toward mothers who were punitive or disapproving of the children's activity.

Riojas-Cortez (2000) observed that when Mexican American children had the opportunity to engage in sociodramatic play, the richness of their language was revealed in their play. The preschoolers were able to create elaborate monologues and dialogues in their native language, and in some cases their second language as well.

Tenenbaum and Leaper (1997) found that both Mexican American mothers and fathers asked more questions overall during feminine-stereotyped play than during masculine-stereotyped play. Parent–child pairs were asked to play with three different toy sets: First, a toy zoo set consisting of plastic zoo animals and fences, which was a gender-neutral toy for warm-up; second, there was a toy set consisting of plastic plates, pots and pans, and food, which was considered feminine stereotyped; the third toy set was a track set consisting of a track requiring assembly and trains, which were considered masculine stereotyped. The study was a naturalistic one carried out in the family's home with an observer. Results found that egalitarian fathers asked more questions than the more traditional fathers during the toy food play, with gender attitude having a large effect size. For mothers, the gender of the child was a significant predictor of their total questions. Also, the language spoken was a significant predictor of the proportion of conceptual questions asked. English-speaking mothers were more likely than Spanish-speaking mothers to use conceptual questions during the toy food play. In summary, both mothers and fathers asked more questions during the feminine-stereotyped toy food play than the masculine-stereotyped toy track play. Fathers were more cognitively demanding than mothers with their children, stimulating the child's cognitive development. The fathers of Mexican descent were less interested in focusing on teaching concepts and more interested in simply playing, whereas the mothers may have been more concerned with challenging their children's thinking, in particular asking more questions of their sons than daughters than the fathers (Tenenbaum & Leaper, 1997).

Leaper (2000) looked further at gender, affiliation, and assertion between parent and child play with 98 U.S. children 3–5 years of age with their parents of European, Latin American, or multiethnic backgrounds. The mothers and fathers were separately videotaped in their home while interacting with their child under the same set play conditions as Tenenbaum and Leaper (1997). Overall, mothers and fathers, regardless of culture, were more interactive and engaged with their child during the toy food play than during the use of the toy track and train. In addition, fathers were more assertive than mothers with their child, and the children tended to demonstrate higher assertion levels with mothers than with fathers.

Cross-culturally, Latino child–parent pairs demonstrated significantly higher levels of connectedness and affiliation than either European American or mixed-ethnicity child–parent pairs during the toy track and train activity. The Latino children in turn also demonstrated significantly higher affiliation and connection than European American or mixed-ethnicity children (Leaper, 2000). Thus, it appears that Latino families tended to express both more assertion and under certain circumstances more affiliation than non-Latino families. These findings appear consistent with reports that Mexican and other Latin American families emphasize family closeness (Bornstein, Haynes, Pascual, Painter, & Galperin, 1999; Gaines, Buriel, Liu, & Rios, 1997). Therefore, play therapists need to be aware that social collaborative play may have different meanings and serve different functions depending on the family's sociocultural background.

Toys, Games, and Types of Play

Many of the games played by Mexican American adults as a child are slowly fading away from the culture and are being lost to the current generations of children. Games were taught to the young by their mothers and their grammar school teachers, who in turn had learned them from their own mothers and teachers. Mexican American families have little time to teach their children the games of the past that reflect their culture (Castillo, 2004). Many Mexican American parents struggle to keep themselves financially stable, often requiring both parents to work long hours, thereby leaving their children to be cared for by a babysitter or daycare provider. When the parents get home in the evening, household chores, preparing dinner, and getting ready for the next day occupy their time, while their children watch television or play among themselves. These parents remember the times when they played *escondidas*, or *el bote* (tin can). *El bote* involves a person being "it," taking the can and slamming it down on the curb. Another child then kicks the can out into the street as far as possible. The child who is "it" races to retrieve the can and runs back to slam it down on the curb. In the meantime, all the other children run to find a hiding place. The child who retrieved the can then goes to look for the children, and once another is found the race is on between them to reach the can and slam it to the curb first in order to be safe. The "loser" is then "it," and the game begins anew (Castillo, 2004).

El chicote (the whip) was another favorite. The children face opposite directions, clasp each other's wrists, and the lead person of this chain runs as fast as possible, with the group of children holding on for dear life. As the group runs in a serpent-like fashion, the last person in the chain gets the most action and often would be half-running and half-flying in the air. Not all games were as physically active, however. Children would play marbles or manipulate a yo-yo.

The game *el balero* demanded more skill and concentration. It was played with a toy made of two wooden pieces tied loosely together by a string. The goal was to swing the larger round piece of wood by the string and hook it onto the cylindrical piece of wood. *Loteria*, or lottery, was a card game. Everyone had to memorize the names of a series of nouns on each card. This game gave the family an opportunity to spend an enjoyable evening together before bedtime.

Many girls spent time indoors dressing their *munecas* (dolls), while the boys, and some girls, were busy outside with their *rompos* (tops). The boys needed strength to make the wooden tops spin off a string onto the ground. The boy who could spin his top the longest was the winner.

Other cultural games included making roads in the dirt with a stick and using the imagination to make bridges and trains out of pieces of cardboard, using bottle caps as wheels. Many children in Mexico did not have store-bought toys. In contrast to today, expensive toys have fast replaced these simple toys and games, losing some of the natural creativity along the way. Compared to the games that children used to play in Mexico, today's toys and games lack the vitality, imagination, and innocence of traditional Hispanic games. These cultural games also helped to teach children the important socialization skills needed to live in any society. Often the children would come in early to start a game, and then continue it throughout the day during recess and even after school before going home (Castillo, 2004).

The demands of the society on the family is in part responsible for the disappearance of traditional Mexican games. Mexican American families have found it necessary to trade of their Hispanic culture to stay within mainstream society (Castillo, 2004).

Mexico

Parent–Child Interaction

Mayan parents in rural Yucatan, Mexico, an agriculturally based economy, are heavily engaged in work. The culture gives priority to adult activities and work; children are left to negotiate their way through it with minimal disruption by paying attention to what is going on all the time, making sense of activities as best as possible, and learning through watching (Gaskins, 2000).

Children are expected not to interrupt or get in the way, and to contribute to the household work as needed and able (Gaskins, 2000). Cultural understandings about the world help shape a child's experiences. "There are many health concerns for Mayan parents of young children, stemming from environmental hazards, characteristics of the body, and supernatural dangers" (Gaskins, 2000, p. 379). The Maya believe that children develop from internal preprogramming that occurs naturally and is continual. They do not monitor the progress of a child's development or create experiences that will improve or hasten it. By age 5, children are expected to take responsibility for personal bathing, dressing, grooming, eating, and sleeping. The children are highly independent and competent in self-care, with little or no pressure or encouragement from the parents. Although involved in adult-directed work activities, they are expected to find things to do independently when not occupied. Parents offer little direction to influence children's behavior, including when to start school or how much to sleep and eat, allowing their children a greater range of independence in general (Gaskins, 2000). The children spend their early years carefully observing their environment, parental activities and work, and the community's activities until they know these by heart.

Although there is much social contact, there is little social interaction, especially with adults. Young children do not initiate conversations with adults unless a very specific request is needed. In turn, the adults rarely speak to the children unless it is to have them do or not do something specific. The children are more likely to talk to one another within the same age group, but there are often long periods of silence. Such lack of contact may look like withdrawal or lack of engagement to a mainstream U.S. observer (Gaskins, 2000).

Children will play according to their own agenda, with almost no adult interference or support. However, in general, play is not supported as a children's activity by parents, because it is seen as competing with the adult work activities. It is tolerated when it helps to occupy them and seen as an indication that the children are not sick, but discouraged when it directly conflicts with the adults' or children's work. All children older than 1½ or 2 years are expected to do whatever chores they are asked to efficiently and quickly. The parental view is that working and doing chores will help the children to grow into competent and motivated workers, and thus will reflect their responsible parenting (Gaskins, 2000). Other researchers have also reported that Mexican mothers attach no particular value to play and likewise do not believe that it is important to play with their children (Bornstein et al., 1999; Farver, 1993).

Toys, Games, and Types of Play

In the Yucatan, Mayan infants (up to age 2) spend most of their time in large motor and manipulative play, with social, verbal, or symbolic play rare. Play is a dominant activity for children 3–5 years of age, taking almost 40% of the time. Play is divided between objects and large motor play, with little of it symbolic or pretend play (Gaskins, 2000). Older children (aged 6–11) will organize spontaneous pretend play, assigning specific roles to younger children and enacting scenarios from adult life, such as playing house, hunting, or driving to Cancun to sell produce (Gaskins, 2000).

Edwards (2000) found that in Juxtlahuaca, a farming community of low SES, older girls were most responsible for child care. The younger children were kept inside their courtyards with supervising adults who did not stimulate or encourage play, but were tolerant and noncritical. While children ran errands for the adults, they would engage in unstructured play. There were also often games with rules, such as tag and ball, along with playing with dolls and other toys. In addition, children frequently used role play and creative/constructive play—especially the girls, who would pretend to make houses, sew, and prepare tortillas. They would also dig in the sand, use old bricks in numerous ways, and play with pieces of palm and cloth. The boys would have top-spinning contests, play with toy cars, and make roads and vehicles out of mud. No fantasy play was noticed.

PLAY IN NATIVE AMERICAN/INDIGENOUS CULTURES

There is no *one* Native American culture, but a collection of diverse cultures. There are over 500 recognized tribes in the United States, with every tribe different from the rest in some aspects, while similar in others. However, certain core or root themes appear to underlie traditions of Native American and other indigenous North American cultures (e.g., the Eskimo or Inuit culture of Alaska and northern Canada). One of the values most frequently associated with these cultures is the pervasive belief in the sacredness of life, where religious experience is constant and surrounds the individual at all times (Jostad, McAvoy, & McDonald, 1996; McDonald & McAvoy, 1997). There is a clear, reciprocal, and interdependent relationship with all of creation, and humans are inseparable from nature. The Inuit, for example, speak of humans and animals as equal members of a shared environment (Stairs & Wenzel, 1992).

There is also a belief in the cyclical or circular pattern of life, which in turn is recreated at every level of the culture (architecture, dance, music, religion, sports, art, games, and other play) (McDonald & McAvoy, 1997). Another important component is the importance of the spoken word (Beck, Walters, & Francisco, 1992). Thinking before speaking is expected. This thoughtful pause has often been interpreted by European Americans as withdrawal, or stereotyped as a characteristic of stoic and silent people. "Sacred knowledge is often passed down in oral forms, in contrast to Christian religion's emphasis on the written word. Elders are repositories of this oral knowledge" (McDonald & McAvoy, 1997, p. 150).

There is also a wide variety of Native American/indigenous games and other types of play, too numerous to list. Games may be divided into four general categories: (1) games of kinetic competence and dexterity, (2) games of chance, (3) games of representation, and (4) games of strategy (Roberts, Arth, & Bush, 1959). Games of chance were created to develop risk taking, competition, and the power of observation. Games of dexterity were designed to develop stamina, strength, dexterity, and speed. These classes of games are found in over 130 Native American tribes with over 30 different linguistic stocks (Fletcher, 1915), even in the most widely separated ones (Schroeder, 1995). Early tribal games were used as a means to enhance skills needed for the hard work of hunting, planting, gathering, and fighting for survival. Many have been modified through contact with European Americans (Cheska, 1979). Many popular contemporary sports have their origins in indigenous games, such as lacrosse, field hockey, soccer, football, baseball, bowling, sled-dog racing, running, swimming, throwing spears (javelins), shooting arrows, wrestling, and racquetball. However, not much credit or recognition has been given to the indigenous groups that developed the early versions of these sports (Schroeder, 1995). Current play interactions appear to lack the degree of competitiveness seen in European American culture. Winning and losing are largely irrelevant (Farrer, 1990). There are subtle differences between how a group of Native American youth play a basketball game and how European American youth do: "Native Americans often seem to concentrate more on playing the game well rather than putting down an opponent. They also often make subtle adjustments in the rules to accommodate their definition and style of competition" (McDonald & McAvoy, 1997, p. 152). Successful Native American women "view competition differently than 'mainstream' society. They look at competition as a motivating, stimulating force that spurs groups as well as individuals toward greatness" (Schroeder, 1995, p. 49).

Characteristics of play in a few indigenous cultures are now described.

Apache Culture

Parent–Child Interaction

Over 2,100 people appear on the tribal rolls as official Mescalero Apaches who live on a reservation in south central New Mexico. There are two major dialects of Apachean spoken at Mescalero, Mescalero and Chiricahua, as well as several other languages (Lipan, English, Spanish, and Navajo). Language is important at Mescalero, as it identifies kin, ancestry, and length of time on the reservation. Children tend to speak the dialect of their mothers, through whom relational ties are strongest (Farrer, 1990).

Four organizing principles are basic to Mescalero world order: balance, the number four, silence, and circularity (Farrer, 1990). The use of circles is an important cultural component, with traditional homes, dances, communication, and play all having a circular arrangement, and most movement occurring in a clockwise fashion. "The rule of speaking in clockwise turns is so strong that it can be seen in operation even during rather heated arguments. Balance is believed to exist in that no one dominates conversation" (Farrer, 1990, p. 124).

Parents are rarely noted to correct their children in a public setting. However, children are expected to behave appropriately, having observed parents, older siblings, and other relatives. Minor misbehavior is ignored. If it should be more serious, then a child is physically restrained or may be removed from the situation (Farrer, 1990). If a parental look does not stop the child's behavior, then an older sibling or relative will go to attend to the child, and consequences will be dealt with in the privacy of the home.

Mescalero Apaches are not more stoic or less feeling than European Americans: "It is simply impolite to express emotions in public. They are silent on personal matters, especially those of an emotional nature" (Farrer, 1990, p. 51). People are considered unsocialized or not themselves if they express emotions in public, and doing so is a cause for embarrassment if outsiders are present. Although Mescaleros are great teasers and jokers among their intimates, such behavior is considered grossly impolite in the presence of strangers. Moreover, anger, grief, or sadness are never permitted in public; these are seen as the most private of emotions, along with expressions of love (Farrer, 1990).

The Apachean belief system emphasizes harmony and balance between this world and the supernatural one. One is to move through life and on earth disturbing as little as possible, so that words and speech, as well as actions, can be a disturbance. Questioning is done indirectly through statements rather than through direct inquiries. Direct questions are not to be asked in personal matters, although they are avoided even in nonpersonal ones. During council meetings, all have an opportunity to talk, with the eldest in a family speaking first and speaking for the entire family. Each speaker is given as much time as necessary, with no one being interrupted. In social situations, relatives speak to each other more often and in more depth than with nonrelatives.

Mescalero Apache people find it essential to be close to persons with whom they are interacting. Closeness is both security and an indication of willingness to interact. Often people will touch each other when engaged in conversation, standing side by side with their upper arms touching. When several people talk together, the group appears in a tight formation with no room for another to join, but will expand to include another.

Personal space is much closer for Mescalero Apaches than it is for European Americans. Touching during social occasions is considered to be comfortable and polite rather than carrying a sexual message, as it does in European American society (Farrer, 1990).

It is easy for miscommunication to occur between European American teachers and Mescalero Apache children, as children crowd around their teachers and each other in classrooms, hallways, and the cafeteria. Farrer (1990) gives an example: An Apache child had invaded a teacher's personal space with her body contact. The teacher maintained contact with her hand, but moved her body out of contact. The Apache child felt rejected, since the teacher refused to allow body contact; the teacher felt that the child had not been admitted to the conversation, since no eye contact had been made. For children, the normal way of communicating "is by standing close to the side of the person with whom you are engaged in conversation . . . people's eyes are usually straight ahead or cast down and their bodies do not move until the interaction is terminated" (Farrer, 1990, p. 89).

Toys, Games, and Types of Play

Farrer (1990) has described a Mescalero version of tag, *nedit*, with children running from the others, saying "not it," or trying to tag one another. Verbal interaction among the children is minimal, even if a player is making a mistake. There is no verbal correction, although much vocalizing of feelings and reactions occurs. If a child does not play properly, the game will just stop, or the children will just not play with that person again. Mescalero tag is not linear but circular; it is played using a jungle gym, with the children (unusual for Mescalero culture) moving counterclockwise. A person becomes "it" when deliberately touched on the head, shoulder, arm, or leg.

Additional games include horseback races and other games, baseball, basketball, foot races, and jacks, as well as made-up games of climbing trees and fences, rock throwing, and jumping steps. Rock throwing is a boys' activity with the intent to throw a rock against a moving target. It is not hostile, but rather becomes a game of concentration, dexterity, and skill. Solitary play is rare and seldom occurs (Farrer, 1990). Jacks, usually a girls' game, is played in silence. The girls play sitting close to one another, with others watching. Turns move clockwise, and when a girl makes a mistake, she collects the jacks and passes them to the girl on her left without conversation.

The children prefer to play with relatives over nonrelatives. Children who are within a kinship group usually play together more often than they include or join in with nonrelatives. Frequently teams of relatives will join each other for a game. Winning and losing are largely irrelevant, with no score kept in football or in any of the other games. The importance is in the playing, and in doing so well and properly—and, if possible, cooperatively (Farrer, 1990).

Eskimo/Inuit Culture

The village of Tununak on Nelson Island, along the Bering Sea coast of Alaska, still retained much of its culture and way of life at the time when it was studied by Ager (1977). Hunting and fishing supplied the staples of the diet, and the people still all spoke Yupik, their native tongue. The culture was notable for its lack of rigid, formal, hierarchical social relationships, with an emphasis on equal standards of living for everyone and a lack of formal authority in leaders.

Ager (1977) found that games of physical skill and memory/attention were overwhelmingly preferred to other types, as dexterity, strength, endurance, and sharp mental abilities were functional in a society dependent upon these qualities in both its male and female members. Self-reliance and independence were other valued personal traits, and thus individual self-testing games such as "story knifing" and making string figures were very popular. Competition was minimized, with everyone trying to do their best, but not at the others' expense. It was consistent with cultural views that one person's gain is not necessarily another's loss. During game nights organized for the children, no prizes were given out for telling the best stories or for making the quickest string figures. The high value placed on nonaggression within the group was reflected "in the lack of malice in games and sports among the Eskimos . . . participants do not become angry at one another . . . losers are good sports. They leave laughing" (Ager, 1977, p. 95). However, laughter was not always an indication of amusement; it could be a means of concealing shame or hurt feelings.

There was little emphasis in games upon equipment; for instance, a version of baseball was played with any handy piece of wood. There was also no provision in playing for winning another's possessions, such as in playing marbles. All players left with their own marbles. The enjoyment was in the contest of skill, not in taking another's marbles as a prize (Ager, 1977). With increased European American contact and the resulting new materials, games of strategy (chess, checkers), games combining chance and strategy (board games, card games), and sports such as basketball and football (combining physical skill and strategy) were adopted by the children and adults.

UNIVERSAL ASPECTS OF PLAY

Despite the diversity of play in different cultures, various aspects of children's play appear universal. First and foremost, play is integrally related to other major characteristics of all cultures, such as religion, levels of sub-sistence, social complexity, and child-rearing customs.

The categories of games played across cultures seem to be consistent: games of physical skill, strategy, problem solving, memory/attention, and chance (Chick, 1998). The inclusion of only some or all these types of games in a culture reflects the level of cultural complexity. No culture lacks games of physical skill, whereas games of chance do not occur in all cultures (Chick, 1998). The nature of children's play across cultures can also be re-duced to four major types: (1) play as imitation of and/or preparation for adult life, (2) play as a game or sports activity for physical skill, (3) play as a projective or an expressive activity, and (4) play as a pastime. In particu-lar, some forms of children's play in all cultures can be characterized as being imitative or mimicking the activities of the adult world. It appears that this type of play occurs in anticipation of adult life, with children re-hearsing and learning the necessary components in growing complexity as they mature (Schwartzman & Barbera, 1977). Furthermore, the types and extent of play are universally related to particular types of child-rearing practices. Even in cultures that put children to work with chores and eco-nomically based activities at an early age, the children play during free time or entwine play with the course of the work/chore.

Many games themselves are common across all peoples. The Interna-tional Council on Health, Physical Education, and Recreation (1967) listed more than 65 different games and 39 dances from 58 countries. Games played across cultures include variations of jacks, certain sports, variations of tag (or "it"), kite flying, and card games. Although specific rules or other aspects of games can vary from culture to culture, a game cannot begin until the rules are agreed on, learned, and followed. Children across all cultures are also creative and innovative in using natural and environmen-tal materials to create toys and props for their games and other forms of play.

In addition, gender emerges as a significant factor. Boys tend to play more often in an exploratory mode, whereas girls play more often in a symbolic mode, regardless of culture (Bornstein et al., 1999). Mothers of boys engage in more exploratory play, and mothers of girls engage in more symbolic play across cultures. There has also been evidence of socioeco-nomic and other cultural differences in the extent to which children en-gage in dramatic and sociodramatic play; however, it appears that these forms of play occur naturally at about the same age in all young children, regardless of their SES or other cultural characteristics (Griffing, 1974). Finally, socioeconomic factors play a significant part in both environmen-tal intellectual advantage and play-oriented activities. A positive signifi-cant correlation was found between higher SES and an intellectually more advantageous family environment, regardless of race or of whether a child was born preterm or full-term (Gottfried, 1986). And middle- and upper-SES parents, in contrast to low-SES parents, make available a greater amount of play materials and are more involved with their children, particularly in play-oriented activities (Gottfried, 1986).

CONCLUSION

It is readily apparent that the numbers of children and families from culturally diverse backgrounds are increasing rapidly in the United States. As U.S. society becomes more culturally pluralistic, it is essential for us to become more aware of and sensitized to the cultural differences among the children we work with, and to help children embrace these differences. Awareness of differences in others' language, skin color, or customs is seen by age 3, along with the beginning of stereotyping (Rettig, 2002). We also need to develop strategies to utilize these differences, rather than making the children accommodate themselves to mainstream U.S. culture. It is important to remember that other cultures may not use verbal means for learning (the predominant European American mode of teaching), but rather modeling and observational skills. In addition, a period of silence or a long pause may not signal a lack of attention or language problems, but perhaps a cultural norm for communication. Similarly, close physical proximity may be a necessity for communication and play, rather than an intrusion into personal space. Other examples come readily to mind. In many Native American and Asian cultures, for instance, it is inappropriate for children to make eye contact with their elders during communication; this is in marked contrast to mainstream U.S. culture, where eye contact shows attentiveness and respect. A child from a Native American background may resent being touched, especially on the head or hair, because in that culture only certain relatives may touch one's head. And Native American children may prefer not to ask a lot of questions, preferring to watch and observe in order to learn (Rettig, 2002). Game-playing and sitting styles are circular in many cultures (e.g., among the Mescalero Apaches, as described earlier).

Lack of competitiveness, or cheating in games, may be a cultural factor rather than a signal of a potential problem. Cultural differences can also play out in language, social interactions, and methods of child rearing, all of which can easily be misunderstood and cause problems. As professionals, we need to be alert for whatever we might say that conveys a value judgment. We must understand the cultural diversity of the children we work with by seeking out information regarding ethnicity and other cultural characteristics of the neighborhood and families, and the cultural meaning and significance of the children's play. The most valuable information can come from observing and talking with individuals representing different cultural groups, and from participating in their family events and celebrations. Finally, one of the best ways of promoting and obtaining cultural awareness of play is through the use of play itself!

REFERENCES

Ager, L. P. (1977). The reflection of cultural values in Eskimo children's games. In D. F. Lancy & B. A. Tindall (Eds.), *The study of play: Problems and prospects* (pp. 92–98). West Point, NY: Leisure Press.

Allison, M.T. (1992). Sport, culture and socialization. In M. T. Allison (Ed.), *Play, leisure and quality of life: Social scientific perspectives* (pp. 211–232). Dubuque, IA: Kendall/Hunt.

Avellar, J., & Kagan, S. (1976). Development of competitive behaviors in Anglo-American and Mexican-American children. *Psychological Reports, 39,* 191–198.

Barnett, L. A. (1990). Developmental benefits of play for children. *Journal of Leisure Research, 22*(2), 138–153.

Barta, J., & Schaelling, D. (1998). Games we play: Connecting mathematics and culture in the classroom. *Teaching Children Mathematics, 4*(7), 388–393.

Beck, P., Walters, A., & Francisco, N. (1992). *The sacred: Ways of knowledge, sources of life.* Tsaile, AZ: Navajo Community College Press.

Begley, S. (1996, February 19). Your child's brain. *Newsweek,* pp. 55–59.

Bellah, R. N., Madsen, R., Sullivan, W. M., Swindler, A., & Tipton, S. M. (1985). *Habits of the heart: Individualism and commitment in American life.* New York: Harper & Row.

Bloch, M. N., & Pellegrini, A. D. (1989). Ways of looking at children, context and play. In M. N. Bloch & A. D. Pellegrini (Eds.), *The ecological context of children's play* (pp. 1–17). Norwood, NJ: Ablex.

Bornstein, M. H. (1994). Cross-cultural perspectives on parenting. In G. d'Ydewalle, P. Eelen, & P. Bertelson (Eds.), *International perspectives on psychological science: Vol. 2. State of the art lectures presented at the XXVth International Congress of Psychology, Brussels, 1992* (pp. 359–369). Hove, UK: Erlbaum.

Bornstein, M. H., Haynes, O. M., Pascual, L., Painter, K. M., & Galperin, C. (1999). Play in two societies: Pervasiveness of process, specificity of structure. *Child Development, 70*(2), 317–331.

Bose, A. B. (1992). *The disadvantaged urban child in India* (Innocenti Occasional Papers). Florence: International Child Development Centre/UNICEF.

Bradley, R. H. (1986). Play materials and intellectual development. In A. W. Gottfried & C. C. Brown (Eds.), *Play interactions: The contribution of play material and parental involvement to children's development* (pp. 227–251). Lexington, MA: Lexington Books.

Bronfenbreener, U. (1979). *The ecology of human development.* Cambridge, MA: Harvard University Press.

Brown, P. S., Sutterby, J. A., Therrell, J. A., & Thornton, C. D. (2000). *The value and contributions of free play to children's development* [Online]. Available at http://www. ipema.org/newrel2.asp

Bruce, T. (1993). The role of play in children's lives. *Childhood Education, 69*(4), 237–238.

Bunker, L. K. (1991). The role of play and motor skill development in building children's self-confidence and self-esteem. *Elementary School Journal, 91*(5), 467–471.

Cady, T. (1996). *Kwanzaa mini-unit* [Online]. Available at http://teacherlink.ed. usu.edu/tlresources/units/Byrnes-celebrations/kwanzaa.html

Castillo, G. (2004). *Traditional Hispanic children's game disappears* [Online]. Available at http://www.epcc.edu/ftp/Homes/monicaw/borderlands/11_traditional_hispanic.htm

Caudill, W., & Weinstein, H. (1969). Maternal care and infant behavior in Japan and America. *Psychiatry, 32*, 12–43.

Cheska, A. T. (1979). Native American games as strategies of societal maintenance. In E. Norbeck & C. R. Farrer (Eds.), *Forms of play of Native North Americans* (pp. 227–247). St. Paul, MN: West.

Chick, G. (1998). Games in culture revisited: A replication and extension of Roberts, Arth, and Bush (1959). *Cross-Cultural Research, 32*(2), 185–206.

Chow, R. (1994). Beyond parental control and authoritarian parenting style: Understanding Chinese parenting through the cultural notion of training. *Child Development, 65*, 1111–1119.

Cook, H., & Chi, C. (1984). Cooperative behavior and locus of control among American and Chinese-American boys. *Journal of Psychology, 118*(2), 169–177.

Donaldson, M. (1978). *Children's minds*. London: Croom Helm.

Duncan, G., Brooks-Gunn, J., & Klebanov, P. (1994). Economic deprivation and early childhood development. *Child Development, 65*, 296–318.

Dunn, J., & Dale, N. (1984). I am daddy: 2-year-olds' collaboration in joint pretend with a sibling and with mother. In I. Bretherton (Ed.), *Symbolic play: The development of social understanding* (pp. 131–158). New York: Academic Press.

Durrett, M. E., O'Bryant, S., & Pennebacker, J. W. (1975). Child-rearing reports of white, black and Mexican American families. *Developmental Psychology, 11*(6), 871–894.

Edwards, C. P. (2000). Children's play in cross-cultural perspective: A new look at the Six Cultures Study. *Cross-Cultural Research, 34*(4), 318–338.

Eisert, D., & Lamorey, S. (1996). Play as a window on child development: The relationship between play and other developmental domains. *Early Education and Development, 7*(3), 221–234.

Eisner, E. W. (1990). The role of art and play in children's cognitive development. In E. Klugman & S. Smilansky (Eds.), *Children's play and learning: Perspectives and policy implications* (pp. 43–56). New York: Teachers College Press.

Ericksen, J. A., Yancey, W. L., & Ericksen, E. P. (1979). The division of family roles. *Journal of Marriage and the Family, 41*, 301–313.

Erikson, E. (1963). *Childhood and society* (rev. ed.). London: Routledge & Kegan Paul.

Farrer, C. R. (1990). *Play and inter-ethnic communication: A practical ethnography of the Mescalero Apache*. New York: Garland Press.

Farver, J. (1993). Cultural differences in American and Mexican mother–child pretend play. *Merrill–Palmer Quarterly, 39*(3), 344–356.

Farver, J. (1999). Activity setting analysis: A model for examining the role of culture in development. In A. Goncu (Ed.), *Children's engagement in the world: A sociocultural perspective* (pp. 113–148). Cambridge, UK: Cambridge University Press.

Farver, J., & Shin, Y. (1997). Social pretend play in Korean- and Anglo-American preschoolers. *Child Development, 68,* 544–556.

Farver, J., & Wimbarti, S. (1995). Indonesian children's play with their mothers and older siblings. *Child Development, 66,* 1493–1503.

Feng, J. (1994). *Asian-American children: What teachers should know.* Early Childhood and Parenting Collaborative, Division of Illinois. (ERIC Document Reproduction Service No. ED 369 577)

Fletcher, A. C. (1915). *Indian games and dances with Native songs.* Boston: Stanhope Press.

Fromberg, D. P. (1998). Play issues in early childhood education. In C. Seefeldt (Ed.), *The early childhood curriculum: A review of current research* (2nd ed., pp. 190–212). Columbus, OH: Merrill.

Fromberg, D. P. (2002). *Play and meaning in early childhood education.* Boston: Allyn & Bacon.

Frost, J. L. (1997). Child development and playgrounds. *Parks and Recreation, 32*(4), 54–61.

Frost, J., & Jacobs, P. (1996). Play deprivation and juvenile violence. *Play Rights, 18,* 4.

Gaines, S. O., Jr., Buriel, R., Liu, J. H., & Rios, D. I. (1997). *Culture, ethnicity, and personal relationship processes.* New York: Routledge.

Garbarino, J. (1989). An ecological perspective on the role of play in child development. In M. N. Bloch & A. D. Pellegrini (Eds.), *The ecological context of children's play* (pp. 12–36). Norwood, NJ: Ablex.

Garvey, C. (1977). *Play.* London: Collins/Fontana Open Books.

Gaskins, S. (1996). How Mayan parental theories come into play. In S. Harkness & C. Super (Eds.), *Parents' cultural belief systems* (pp. 345–363). New York: Guilford Press.

Gaskins, S. (1999). Children's daily lives in a Mayan village: a case study of culturally constructed roles and activities. In A. Goncu (Ed.), *Children's engagement in the world: Sociocultural perspectives* (pp. 25–61). Cambridge, UK: Cambridge University Press.

Gaskins, S. (2000). Children's daily activities in a Mayan village: A culturally grounded description. *Cross-Cultural Research, 34*(4), 375–389.

Glover, G. (1999). Multicultural considerations in group play therapy. In D. S. Sweeney & L. E. Homeyer (Eds.), *The handbook of group play therapy* (pp. 278–295). San Francisco: Jossey-Bass.

Goldman, L. R. (1998). *Child's play: Myth, mimesis and make-believe.* New York: Berg.

Goldstein, J. H. (1994). *Toys, play and child development.* Cambridge, UK: Cambridge University Press.

Goncu, A., & Mosier, C. (1991, April). *Cultural variations in the play of toddlers.* Paper presented at the annual meeting of the Society for Research in Child Development, Seattle, WA.

Gottfried, A. W. (1986). The relationships of play materials and parental involvement to young children's cognitive development. In A. W. Gottfried & C. C.

Brown (Eds.), *Play interactions: The contribution of play material and parental involvement to children's development* (pp. 327–333). Lexington, MA: Lexington Books.

Griffing, P. (1974). Sociodramatic play among young black children. *Theory into Practice, 13*(4), 257–265.

Haight, W. (1999). The pragmatics of caregiver-pretending at home: Understanding culturally-specific socialization practices. In A. Goncu (Ed.), *Children's engagement in the world: Sociocultural perspectives* (pp. 128–147). Cambridge, UK: Cambridge University Press.

Haight, W., & Black, J. (2001). A comparative approach to play: Cross-species and cross-cultural perspectives of play in development. *Human Development, 44*, 228–234.

Haight, W., & Miller, P. (1992). The development of everyday pretend play: A longitudinal study of mothers' participation. *Merrill-Palmer Quarterly, 38,* 331–349.

Haight, W. L., & Miller, P. J. (1993). *Pretending at home: Development in sociocultural context.* Albany: State University of New York Press.

Haight, N., Park, R., & Black, J. (1997). Mothers' and fathers' beliefs about spontaneous participations in their toddlers' pretend play. *Merrill-Palmer Quarterly, 42,* 271–290.

Haight, W. L., Wang, X., Fung, H. H., Williams, K., & Mintz, J. (1999). Universal, developmental, and variable aspects of young children's play: A cross-cultural comparison of pretending at home. *Child Development, 70*(6), 1477–1488.

Hammer, C. S., & Weiss, A. (1999). Guiding language development: How African American mothers and their infants structure play. *Journal of Speech, Language and Hearing Research, 42*(5), 1219–1234.

Han, M., & Washington, D. (1988). *Traditional Korean child-rearing practices.* Amherst: University of Massachusetts. (ERIC Document Reproduction Service No. ED 308 945)

Heath, S. B. (1983). *Ways with words: Language, life and work in communities and classrooms.* Cambridge, UK: Cambridge University Press.

Hill, R. (1993). *Research on the African-American family: A holistic perspective.* Westport, CT: Auburn House.

Holland, C., Koblinsky, S., & Anderson, E. A. (1995, July). *Maternal strategies for protecting Head Start children from community violence: Implications for family-focused violence education programs.* Paper presented at the annual meeting of the National Head Start Association, Washington, DC.

Howes, C., & Unger, O. (1989). Play with peers in child care settings. In M. N. Bloch & A. D. Pellegrini (Eds.), *The ecological context of children's play* (pp. 165–190). Norwood, NJ: Ablex.

Hsu, F. L. K. (1961). Kinship and ways of life: An exploration. In F. L. K. Hsu (Ed.), *Psychological anthropology* (pp. 400–456). Homewood, IL: Dorsey Press.

Hughes, F. P. (1999). *Children, play and development.* Needham Heights, MA: Allyn & Bacon.

Huizinga, J. (1949). *Homo ludens.* London: Routledge & Kegan Paul.

Hupp, S. C., Lam, S. F., & Jaeger, J. (1992). Differences in exploration of toys by one-year-old children: A Korean and American comparison. *Behavior Science Research, 26*(1–4), 123–136.

International Council on Health, Physical Education, and Recreation. (1967). *ICHPER book of worldwide games*. Washington, DC: Author.

Isenberg, J. P., & Quisenberry, N. (2003). *Play: Essential for all children*. A position paper of the Association for Childhood Education International. Available at http://www.udel.edu/bateman/acei/playpaper.htm

Jarrett, R., Jefferson, S., & Roach, A. (2000, August). *Family and parenting strategies in high risk African American neighborhoods*. Paper presented at the annual meeting of the National Head Start Association, Washington, DC.

Jostad, P., McAvoy, L., & McDonald, D. (1996). Native American land ethics: Implications for natural resource management. *Society of Natural Resources, 28*(9), 565–581.

Kagan, S. (1978). Social motives and behaviors of Mexican-American and Anglo-American children. In J. L. Martinez (Ed.), *Chicano psychology* (pp. 45–86). New York: Academic Press.

Kagan, S., & Ender, P. B. (1975). Maternal response to success and failure of Anglo-American and Mexican children. *Child Development, 46*, 452–458.

Kearns, B. J. R. (1970). Childrearing practices among selected culturally deprived minorities. *Journal of Genetic Psychology, 116*, 149–155.

Kelly, J. R., & Godbey, G. (1992). *Sociology of leisure*. State College, PA: Venture.

Kim, M. (2002). Parents' perceptions and behavior regarding toys for young children's play in Korea. *Education, 122*(4), 793–808.

Kornadt, H. J., Hayashi, T., Tachibana, Y., Trommsdorff, G., & Yamauchi, H. (1992). Aggressiveness and its developmental conditions in five cultures. In S. Iwawaki, Y. Kashima, & K. Leung (Eds.), *Innovations in cross-cultural psychology* (pp. 250–268). Amsterdam: Swets & Zeitlinger.

Lancy, D. F. (1977). The play behavior of Kpelle children during rapid cultural change. In D. F. Lancy & B. A. Tindall (Eds.), *The study of play: Problems and prospects* (pp. 84–91). West Point, NY: Leisure Press.

Lancy, D. F. (1996). *Playing on the mother-ground: Cultural routines and children's development*. New York: Guilford Press.

Leacock, E. (1976). At play in African villages. In J. S. Bruner, A. Jolly, & K. Sylva (Eds.), *Play: Its role in development and evolution* (pp. 466–473). New York: Basic Books.

Leaper, C. (2000). Gender, affiliation, assertion and the interactive context of parent-child play. *Developmental Psychology, 36*(3), 381–393.

Lebra, T. S. (1976). *Japanese patterns of behavior*. Honolulu: University of Hawaii Press.

Lee, G., & Childress, M. (1999). Promising practices: Playing Korean ethnic games to promote multicultural awareness. *Multicultural Education, 6*(3), 33–35.

Letiecq, B., & Koblinsky, S. A. (2003). *African-American fathering of young children in violent neighborhoods: paternal protective strategies and their predictors* [Online]. Available at http://www.articles.findarticles.com/p/articles/mi_m0PAV/is_3_1/ai_111268931

LeVine, E. S., & Bartz, K. W. (1979). Comparative childrearing attitudes among Chicano, Anglo, and black parents. *Hispanic Journal of Behavioral Sciences, 1*(2), 165–178.

Levin, D. E. (2000). Learning about the world through play. *Early Childhood Today, 15*(3), 56–64.

Martinez, E. A. (1988). Child behavior in Mexican American/Chicano families: Maternal teaching and child-rearing practices. *Family Relations, 37*(3), 275–280.

Martini, M. (1994). Peer interactions in Polynesia: A view from the Marquesas. In J. Roopnarine, J. Johnson, & F. Hooper (Eds.), *Children's play in diverse cultures* (pp. 73–103). Albany: State University of New York Press.

McDonald, D., & McAvoy, L. (1997). Native Americans and leisure: State of the research and future directions. *Journal of Leisure Research, 29*(2), 145–167.

Miller, P., Wiley, A., Fung, H., & Liang, C. (1997). Personal storytelling as a medium of socialization in Chinese and American families. *Child Development, 68*, 557–568.

Mohr, W., Fantuzzo, J., & Abdul-Kabir, S. (2001). Safeguarding themselves and their children: Mothers share their strategies. *Journal of Family Violence, 16*, 75–92.

Monroe, J. E. (1995). Developing cultural awareness through play. *Journal of Physical Education, Recreation and Dance, 66*(8), 24–30.

Moore, T. (1968). Language and intelligence: A longitudinal study of the first eight years. Part II. Environmental correlates of mental growth. *Human Development, 11*, 1–24.

Oke, M., Khattar, A., Pant, P., & Saraswathi, T. S. (1999). A profile of children's play in urban India. *Childhood, 6*(2), 207–219.

Opie, I., & Opie, P. (1988). *The singing games.* New York: Oxford University Press.

Pan, H. W. (1994). Children's play in Taiwan. In J. L. Roopnarine, J. E. Johnson & F. H. Hooper (Eds.), *Children's play in diverse cultures* (pp. 31–50). Albany: State University of New York Press.

Pelligrini, A. D., & Smith, P. K. (1998). Physical activity play: The nature and function of a neglected aspect of play. *Child Development, 69*(3), 577–598.

Piaget, J. (1951). *Play, dreams and imitation in childhood.* New York: Norton.

Quay, L. C., & Pinkett, K. E. L. (1986). Ethnic and social class comparisons of preschoolers' verbal and nonverbal communication in object-centered and object-free play. *Journal of Genetic Psychology, 147*(3), 427–429.

Ramirez, B. A. (1988). Culturally and linguistically diverse children. *Teaching Exceptional Children, 20*(4), 45–46.

Rettig, M. A. (2002). Cultural diversity and play from an ecological perspective. *Children and Schools, 24*(3), 189–199.

Rheingold, H., & Cook, K. V. (1975). The contents of boys' and girls' rooms as an index of parents' behavior. *Child Development, 46*, 459–463.

Riojas-Cortez, M. (2000). Mexican American preschoolers create stories: Sociodramatic play in a dual language classroom. *Bilingual Research Journal, 24*(3), 295–308.

Roberts, J. M., Arth, M. J., & Bush, R. R. (1959). Gamers in culture. *American Anthropologist, 59*, 579–605.

Roopnarine, J., Hossain, Z., Gill, P., & Brophy, H. (1994). Play in the East Indian context. In J. Roopnarine, J. Johnson, & F. Hopper (Eds.), *Children's play in diverse cultures* (pp. 9–30). Albany: State University of New York Press.

Roopnarine, J., & Johnson, J. (1994). A need to look at play in diverse cultural settings. In J. Roopnarine, J. Johnson, & F. Hooper (Eds.), *Children's play in diverse cultures* (pp. 1–8). Albany: State University of New York Press.

Roopnarine, J., Johnson, J., & Hooper, F. (Eds.). (1994). *Children's play in diverse cultures*. Albany: State University of New York Press.

Roopnarine, J. L., Lasker, J., Sacks, M., & Stores, M. (1998). The cultural context of children's play. In O. N. Saracho & B. Spodek (Eds.), *Multiple perspectives on play in early childhood education* (pp. 194–219). Albany: State University of New York Press.

Saloy, M. L. (1999). *African American oral traditions in Louisiana* [Online]. Available at http://www.louisianafolklife.org/LT/Articles_Essays/creole_art_african_am_oral.htm

Sampson, R., Raudenbush, S., & Earls, F. (1997). Neighborhoods and violent crime: A multilevel study of collective efficacy. *Science, 277,* 918–924.

Schroeder, J. J. (1995). Developing self-esteem and leadership skills in Native American women: The role sports and games play. *Journal of Physical Education, Recreation and Dance, 66*(7), 48–52.

Schwartzman, H. B. (1986). A cross-cultural perspective on child-structured play activities and materials. In A. W. Gottfried & C. C. Brown (Eds.), *Play interactions: The Contribution of play materials and parental involvement to children's development* (pp. 13–29). Lexington, MA: Lexington Books.

Schwartzman, H. B., & Barbera, L. (1977). Children's play in Africa and South America: A review of the ethnographic literature. In D. F. Lancy & B. A. Tindall (Eds.), *The study of play: Problems and prospects* (pp. 23–31). West Point, NY: Leisure Press.

Smilansky, S. (1990). Sociodramatic play: Its relevance to behavior and achievement in school. In E. Klugnan & S. Smilansky (Eds.), *Children's play and learning: Perspectives and policy implications* (pp. 18–42). New York: Teachers College Press.

Spodek, B., & Saracho, O. N. (1988). The challenge of educational play. In D. Bergen (Ed.), *Play as a medium for learning and development* (pp. 9–22). Portsmouth, NH: Heinemann.

Stairs, A., & Wenzel, G. (1992). "I am I and the environment": Inuit hunting, community and identity. *Journal of Indigenous Studies, 3*(1), 1–12.

Stevenson, H. W., Stigler, S. L., & Lucker, W. (1985). Cognitive performance and academic achievement of Japanese, Chinese and American children. *Child Development, 56,* 718–734.

Storey, K. S. (1977). Field study: Children's play in Bali. In D. F. Lancy & B. A. Tindall (Eds.), *The study of play: Problems and prospects* (pp. 78–84). West Point, NY: Leisure Press.

Sutton-Smith, B. (1974). The anthropology of play. *Association for the Anthropological Study of Play, 2,* 8–12.

Sutton-Smith, B. (1985). Play research: State of the art. In J. L. Frost & S. Sunderlin (Eds.), *When children play* (pp. 9–16). Wheaton, MD: Association for Childhood Education International.

Sutton-Smith, B. (1986). *Toys as culture*. New York: Gardner Press.

Sutton-Smith, B. (1997). *The ambiguity of play*. Cambridge, MA: Harvard University Press.

Sutton-Smith, B. (1999). Evolving a consilience of play definitions: Playfully. In S. Reifel (Ed.), *Play and culture studies* (Vol. 2, pp. 239–256). Stamford, CT: Ablex.

Sutton-Smith, B., & Roberts, J. M. (1981). Play, games and sports. In H. Triandis & A. Heron (Eds.), *Handbook of cross-cultural psychology: Vol. 4. Departmental psychology* (pp. 425–471). New York: Allyn & Bacon.

Tamis-LeMonda, C. S., Bornstein, M. H., Cyphers, L., Toda, S., & Ogino, M. (1992). Language and play at one year: A comparison of toddlers and mothers in the United States and Japan. *International Journal of Behavioural Development, 15,* 19–42.

Tenenbaum, H. R., & Leaper, C. (1997). Mothers' and fathers' questions to their child in Mexican-Descent Families: Moderators of cognitive demand during play. *Hispanic Journal of Behavioral Sciences, 19*(3), 318–332.

Tobin, J. J., Wu, D. Y. H., & Davidson, D. H. (1989). *Preschool in three cultures.* New Haven, CT: Yale University Press.

Udwin, O., & Shmukler, D. (1981). The influence of sociocultural, economic, and home background factors on children's ability to engage in imaginative play. *Developmental Psychology, 17,* 66–72.

U.S. Bureau of the Census. (1998). *World population profile: 1998.* Retrieved from http://www.census.gov/population/estimates/nation/intfile3-1.txt

Vandermaas-Peeler, M. (2002). Cultural variations in parental support of children's play. In W. J. Lonner, D. L. Dinnel, S. A. Hayes, & D. N. Sattler (Eds.), *Online readings in psychology and culture.* Bellingham: Center for Cross-Cultural Research, Western Washington University. Available at http://www.wwu.edu/~culture)

Vygotsky, L. S. (1967). Play and its role in the mental development of the child. *Soviet Psychology, 17,* 66–72.

Vygotsky, L. S. (1990). Imagination and creativity in childhood. *Soviet Psychology, 28,* 84–96.

Ware, W., & Garber, M. (1972). The home environment as a predictor of school achievement. *Theory into Practice, 11,* 190–195.

Weinberger, L. A., & Starkey, P. (1994). Pretend play by African American children in Head Start. *Early Childhood Research Quarterly, 9,* 327–343.

Weisz, J. R., Rothbaum, F. M., & Blackburn, T. C. (1984). Standing out and standing in: The psychology of control in America and Japan. *American Psychologist, 39,* 955–969.

Whiting, B. B., & Whiting, J. M. W. (1975). *Children of six cultures.* Cambridge, MA: Harvard University Press.

Yeatman, J., & Reifel, S. (1992). Sibling play and learning. *Play and Culture, 5*(2), 141–158.

Zahn-Waxler, C., Friedman, R. J., Cole, P. M., Mizuta, I., & Hiruma, N. (1996). Japanese and United States preschool children's responses to conflict and distress. *Child Development, 67,* 2462–2477.

3

✣

Suggestions and Research on Multicultural Play Therapy

ATHENA A. DREWES

Play is the universal expression of children; it can transcend differences in ethnicity, language, or other aspects of culture. Play can provide the sense of power and control that comes from solving problems and mastering new experiences, ideas, and concerns. It helps build feelings of accomplishment and confidence. Therefore, play therapy is an extremely effective therapeutic intervention to help heal and resolve children's emotional conflicts and issues. This is especially true when play therapists do not have much first-hand knowledge of their clients' cultural characteristics.

As I have noted in Chapter 2, the United States is becoming increasingly culturally diverse. This means that play therapists need to be multiculturally sensitive, so that they can provide the best services to these diverse populations. A play therapist needs to become aware of the various cultural factors affecting each client and family, in order to assess the problem accurately and determine how best to help (Casado & Giblin, 2002). The therapist who makes the effort to learn and know about the symbols, meanings, and impact of a child's culture will be far better able to enter into the child's world through play, and far less likely to make erroneous assumptions that can lead to misdiagnosis and mistreatment. "Cultural differences can affect the validity of assessment as well as the development of therapist–client rapport, therapeutic alliance, and treatment effectiveness" (Schaefer, 1998, p. 4).

Play therapists as a group consider themselves multiculturally competent, even if their training is less than adequate. However, while they rate themselves as most competent in awareness and terminology, they rate themselves as least competent in racial identity and least adequately trained in racial identity (Ritter & Chang, 2002). Many play therapists—especially those who are European Americans—may feel particularly uncomfortable when trying to discuss race and racial differences. Some such therapists may take a "color-blind" approach toward working with clients of other races. They may ignore or avoid race-related content, or disregard the physical appearance or skin color of clients (Kerl, 1999a, 1999b, 1999c). They may feel that a person's race, ethnicity, or other aspects of culture do not matter, and that only the individual is important. But culture does matter! In an attempt not to overgeneralize, some therapists may ignore cultural characteristics completely. This can be harmful in forming the therapeutic alliance, as clients may feel that these therapists are not acknowledging their complete identity. For each individual's culture significantly shapes his or her sense of self, worldview, values, and belief systems (Kerl, 1998). Play therapists who avoid racial issues or ignore the role of culture in other respects may inadvertently contribute to perpetuating unconscious bias. This assumption of a commonality among all individuals—a universality of perspective—may actually mask an unconscious favoritism toward the dominant (European American) culture (Kerl, 2000a, 2000b, 2000c). "If counselors try to ignore or suppress differences based on race, ethnicity, gender and sexual orientation, they will not be able to see their own role in perpetuating bias against these groups" (Kerl, 2000b, p. 11). If the play therapist and client are from different cultural backgrounds, "the practitioner must address the issue of difference in the first session and ask if the clients would prefer to speak with someone from their own ethnic group" (Webb, 2001b, p. 344).

As play therapists, we will all tend to view our clients from our own frame of reference, which can be radically different from our clients'. We must bring this topic up in our intake assessments and throughout treatment (and supervision), rather than risk ignoring it and being viewed by our clients as insensitive (or, worse yet, biased). For example, those of us who are European Americans must overcome our discomfort and be sensitive to the fact that most African Americans have been subjected to much racial prejudice and discrimination. We need to have an understanding of the cultural and racial history of racism, which has resulted in African American clients approaching mental health services with suspicion and hesitancy (Boyd-Franklin, 2003). The play therapist needs to not take their initial reaction personally, which is the challenge in cross-racial work, that of working with a client who may not want to be with you (Boyd-Franklin, 2003).

We must also be sensitive to the fact that Native Americans have over 500 years of ongoing struggle for their land, beliefs, and traditions, and that we have incorporated many stereotypical images (e.g., cowboys and Indians, the Pilgrims and Indians at Thanksgiving) into our cultural view. It is important to assess each client's personal experience of, and degree of identification with, his or her cultural classification. This will only come about through dialogue. We as play therapists need to avoid pathologizing spirituality or religious orientations of our clients. Therapists tend to keep spirituality and religion separate from the work we do in therapy. This is a significant disadvantage in working with many multicultural families who hold strong religious and spiritual beliefs. The use of religion and spirituality in play therapy work can be a powerful joining mechanism with the child and family (Boyd-Franklin, 2003). We do not have to know a lot about their religious or spiritual beliefs, but we can ask with respect and interest, and listen, thereby using it as a strength to join with initially resistant clients who may hold strong beliefs (Boyd-Franklin, 2003).

All of us first need a good grounding in understanding our own personal culture or cultures, and the impact of the culture(s) on us. Our own personal cultural backgrounds, along with our exposure to the dominant culture, lead to the creation of our own worldviews and values. The better we understand the cultural influences on us, the less likely they are to interfere unconsciously with our work. It is important for the play therapist to have self-awareness in order to watch for personal bias and stereotyping, and to be able to examine our own beliefs about families and children (Webb, 2001a). The use of self-assessment questionnaires can help the play therapist understand their own beliefs and views about other cultures (Webb, 2001a). The use of ourselves in the treatment process is what engages clients who are initially hesitant.

However, it is equally important for play therapists not to view clients' race or other cultural factors as the sole reasons behind all their feelings or issues, thereby missing other important variables. Therapists need to be able to distinguish intrapsychic stress from stress created by the social structure. It is important to keep in mind the individualizing impact of ethnic identity development in children in order to avoid overgeneralizing to the culture or stereotyping the problem (Hinman, 2003). Consideration of clients' level of acculturation is critical as well. In particular, play therapists must look into the differences that may occur on an intergenerational level, as issues for recent immigrants may be greater than those for third- or fourth-generation U.S. residents.

Play therapists need to increase their knowledge and understanding of the diverse cultures of their clients. It takes more than reading a book or taking a workshop or two to understand a client's culture; a therapist should research the cultural group, ask questions of the child and family, go to the home for a home visit or in-home therapy session, and (most importantly) attend cultural events and festivals. An understanding of the meaning of play within diverse cultures is also an important factor, along with the inclusion of culturally diverse play materials within the therapist's playroom. Finally, a play therapist should look for a multicultural perspective within supervision to assist with remaining flexible in adjusting to multicultural issues and stances, as well as in treatment planning and progress (Casado & Giblin, 2002). However, the play therapist does not need to know everything about the multiple cultures with which they work (McGoldrick & Giordano, 1996). It would be impossible to do so with the ever-changing nature of culture, how individuals view themselves within the culture with which they identify, and the many variations within each cultural group. Rather, remaining flexible and open to one's own limitations and sharing that with the client is most important. By developing a culturally sensitive practice, the play therapist will help reduce barriers to effective treatment for his or her clients.

POTENTIAL BARRIERS TO MULTICULTURAL WORK, AND SUGGESTED SOLUTIONS

Importance of Family

The play therapist needs to keep in mind how different cultures value the family, and how these values affect the use of play therapy. European American culture values privacy and autonomy, independence, self-care, and egalitarian ideals. In other cultures, family interdependence and family members' caring for each other predominate. "Family" often includes not only the nuclear family, but also extended family members (especially older ones) and close friends. The play therapist needs also to take the child's perspective in seeing who is considered close and influential, instead of assuming that the parents have the primary responsibility for caretaking and nurturing roles (Kerl, 2001). For example, godparents may have more of an influence on a child than blood relatives may. The child may also be developing a cultural identity from their primary caregiver. Additional considerations may arise when the child's ethnic identity is being developed by parents who come from two different cultures. The child then has to face integrating these two cultures, one of which may be a dominant culture. The child's struggle to adjust, and desire, to belong to the dominant culture can place them at odds with being different from their family members and lead to problems in joining effectively with their peers from other cultural backgrounds (Hinman, 2003).

African Americans

African American families have a strong sense of family and a positive racial identity (Forehand & Kotchick, 1996). There is great loyalty to the family, reinforced through community pressure that everything a person does reflects on the family. People are respected not for successes, but for their intrinsic worth; moreover, no person succeeds for self alone, but for family and race (Glover, 1999). Elderly persons are revered, especially women. There is a strong reliance on religion and church for guidance. Children may voice opinions, but not argue with adults once a decision has been made (Hines, Garcia-Preto, McGoldrick, Almedia, & Weltman, 1992). Strong and sometimes harsh discipline is used to teach children which behaviors are acceptable, and children are expected to obey and respect adults. Grooming and appearance are important. Both verbal and nonverbal forms of communication are used, and hands-on experiences are often preferred. African American children may be more boisterous than other children. Religion and spirituality are held in importance. Elders, especially the matriarchs of the family, are respected and may hold important roles in whether or not the treatment will succeed (Boyd-Franklin, 2003).

Asian Americans

Asian cultures value only behaviors that maintain home and family. The individual is valued, but within the context of the family, and bringing praise and honor to the family is a primary goal. It is expected that the individual will make personal sacrifices for the good of the family (Glover, 1999). Asian Americans have a strong ethnic identity, with self-respect, self-control, dignity, and humility valued. Respect is given to older members by virtue of their maturity. Parents expect their children to repress strong emotions in obedience to parental authority and family honor. Independence and self-directedness may be viewed as aggressiveness and stubbornness. Children are expected to work hard and excel academically.

Asian American children's names are carefully chosen as to provide a connection with the family. With adult Asian American clients their title and last name should be used, while using a child's first name is appropriate (Vargas & Koss-Chioino, 1992). However, therapists should avoid using their first name with Asian American clients and parents (Hinman, 2003). Rather, the play therapist should use their title and last name, which would indicate the therapist's strong ties to their own family (Vargas & Koss-Chioino, 1992).

Establishing privacy and confidentiality with Japanese American clients is critical due to their feelings of shame and failure as parents in seeking help for a mental health problem for their children. Setting up and clarifying the structure of the therapy process and relationship and the play therapist's commitment to confidentiality is important. It allows for the therapist to show respect for the shame they feel and allows for these issues to be revisited later on in the process (Hinman, 2003).

Cambodian American and Vietnamese may view a request for help as creating a debt that the family is compelled to pay (Huang, 1998). The play therapist needs to communicate their credibility as a professional and the credibility of play therapy as a treatment intervention (Hinman, 2003). Through such an active exchange of concerns and thoughts, the issue of credibility can be resolved and the client able to trust that the play therapist can be of help to their child (Hinman, 2003).

Hispanic Americans

The strength of the Hispanic family is a primary value, with strong family ties maintained over generations. Parents, especially mothers, expect to have close relationships with their children. Mothers and daughters are expected to develop reciprocal relationships in adulthood, and eldest sons are often expected to provide financial support to older parents (Glover, 1999). Behaviors that encourage family closeness, respect for parental authority, and interpersonal relatedness are fostered. Religion is a great source of strength for many Hispanic families. Psychological problems may be described in physical terms, such as "nerves" or a "stomachache" (Glover, 1999). (See "Culturally Bound Syndromes," below.)

Mexican American families may focus on "personalismo," the personal contact, attention, warmth, and genuineness of the therapist in joining with them (Ramirez, 1998). A warm handshake and close proximity with a Mexican American parent can help to lessen anxiety over seeking help for their child (Hinman, 2003). Mexican American families may also prefer a more directive therapist, deferring to authority and not openly questioning conclusions they may disagree with (Ramirez, 1998). Consequently, premature termination of treatment may occur with the play therapist not understanding why. The therapist needs to repeatedly encourage the Mexican American client to ask questions and state their reactions to the treatment process (Hinman, 2003) in order to avoid barriers.

Native Americans

Native Americans, though a heterogeneous group, do strongly value increased attention to the family and to ongoing family relationships. "Family" includes the extended family, and there is a heightened respect for elders. In addition, the values of sharing, cooperation, and harmony with nature are strong in many tribes (Kerl, 2000a). Children refer to many significant adults as "aunt" and "uncle," and all elders may be referred to as "grandmother" or "grandfather." Parenting styles are permissive, with value placed on independence and abundant opportunities to make choices. Children are not punished often; instead, reasoning is used to show

how the bad behavior affects others. Embarrassment is also used to correct negative behaviors (Glover, 1999).

Issues of Privacy, Trust, and Beliefs

Communication difficulties between therapists or school personnel and culturally different students may be exacerbated when the children are troubled. Families from various cultures may be reluctant to disclose and discuss family problems, to "air their dirty laundry in public," that affect their children's functioning or academic performance. Hispanic, Asian, and Native American families are often reluctant to discuss family problems; all these cultures place a high value on the privacy of family matters (Cochran, 1996). In Asian and Hispanic cultures, if a negative diagnosis is involved, the family will want the client shielded from the news and will prefer that outsiders not be told. Strong adherence to stoicism, fears of deportation, and cultural loyalty may also be contributing factors. Consequently, if a family is reluctant to disclose or discuss difficulties, a child in turn may not wish to reveal material during the course of play therapy. Consultation with a religious leader or family elder, or inclusion of such a person in the treatment discussions, may help to lessen concerns about privacy. In some cultures, such as many traditional Asian, Hispanic, and Middle Eastern cultures, males are dominant. For clients from these cultures, the play therapist may need to consider not just asking mothers or other female family members to make decisions regarding treatment, but fathers or other male relatives as well.

Families from some cultures may see mental health services as either irrelevant or oppressive, because they only come in contact with mental health professionals when forced to by the courts, by welfare agencies, or by other governmental agencies. Therefore, their past experiences may be negative, and they may be reluctant to accept counseling services (Kalish-Weiss, 1989). Recent immigrants may be in need of treatment but reluctant to accept it for many reasons: disillusionment over the difference between their fantasies or expectations and the reality of life in America; marital and familial conflict due to changes in roles; financial difficulties; discrimination; and increased mental health problems due to acculturative stress (Saldana, 2001). Moreover, oppression and trauma experienced in their home countries before immigration can affect families' sense of vulnerability, trust in others, and behaviors to such an extent that they may appear paranoid (Saldana, 2001). Native Americans experience much stress on reservation lands—marginalization and discrimination, along with overall high rates of alcohol and drug use, high suicide and homicide rates, and high rates of child abuse and neglect (Kerl, 2000a). They are severely limited in their access to mental health services; may not be aware of the resources that do exist; and tend to underutilize mental health services in any case because of fear, mistrust, and insensitivity by counselors to their values and needs (Kerl, 2000a).

Diverse cultures contain varying beliefs about what is considered "illness"; what causes the illness (physical imbalance, the ill will of others, or God as punishment for sin); what should be done to promote healing (some cultures may feel that treatment will have little effect or that *curanderos*, or folk healers, are indicated); and what the desired outcome should be. Play therapists should not assume that clients' views match their own, or that normal behavior is the same for everyone regardless of social, cultural, economic, or political background (Coleman, Parmer, & Barker, 1993). Instead, therapists should ask clients and their families what they think caused their problems, respect religious beliefs, learn about the beliefs and practices of the clients' culture, and keep in mind that there are individual variations within cultural groups.

Failure to understand clients' and families' beliefs can cause them to lose trust in the play therapist. For example, innocently complimenting a child without taking proper measures to counteract *mal de ojo*, or the "evil eye," is believed by many cultures to cause the child to become ill with severe headache, uncontrollable weeping, fretfulness, insomnia, or fever (Falicov, 1998) due to implied jealousy. Some Mexicans require touching a child when complimenting him or her; some Ethiopians and Greeks require spitting at the child; and some Filipinos/Filipinas require making the sign of the cross on the child's forehead with one's saliva. Various amulets to ward off the "evil eye" are worn by Middle Eastern and Mediterranean cultures. As another example, the use of coining and cupping, that is, of putting warm coins or adhering cups or glasses to parts of the body in order to "draw away the sickness," in Asian cultures to raise welts is a traditional medical practice, and not a form of abuse; it is considered to help the body rid itself of toxins.

Asians may hold strong beliefs in fatalism (i.e., the idea that certain challenges and events are preordained), as well as in clear lines defining male and female gender roles. Japanese culture has viewed mental health problems as malingering and therefore willful. Consequently, the parent's failure to resolve such issues and to seek outside assistance represents a failure in parenting (Hinman, 2003). The number four is avoided in some Asian and Native American cultures, as it signifies death. Native Americans may follow traditional preferences for explaining natural phenomena according to the supernatural. They also accord great importance to traditional rituals and sacraments, although spiritual beliefs and practices can vary across the over 500 recognized tribes in the United States. It is generally believed that if one breaks with tradition, the resulting disharmony would show through disease, distress, or disability (Lewis & Hayes,

1991). Each tribe may have its own strong beliefs, such as the Navajo taboo on discussing relatives who have died (Glover, 1999).

Religion may also play an important part in a client's family and the culture; if so, it needs to be honored and discussed. Home and traditional remedies may be strongly believed in and used.

Culturally Related Syndromes

Play therapists should be aware that they may encounter various culturally related syndromes, either in family histories or as presenting problems. Saldana (2001) and Falicov (1998) have highlighted some of them:

- *Amok* or *mal de pelea*: Among clients from Malaysia, Laos, the Philippines, Polynesia, Papua New Guinea, and Puerto Rico, a dissociative disorder involving outbursts of violent and aggressive or homicidal behavior directed at people and/or objects.
- *Ataque de nervios*: Among Hispanics, a neurotic or psychotic episode due to a traumatic event; it may include dissociative experiences, hyperkinesis, seizure-like or fainting episodes, mutism, crying spells, or shouting, with possible amnesia for the event afterward.
- *Dhat*: In Indian, Chinese, and Sri Lankan communities, extreme anxiety associated with a sense of weakness and exhaustion.
- *Falling out*: In African American communities, seizure-like symptoms resulting from traumatic events, such as a death in the family.
- *Ghost sickness*: Among Native Americans, weakness and dizziness resulting from the action of witches and evil forces.
- *Hwa-byung*: In Asian communities, pain in the upper abdomen, fear of death, and tiredness resulting from an imbalance between reality and anger.
- *Mal de ojo* (evil eye): Widespread among Mediterranean and Hispanic cultures, more commonly affecting women and children; it is believed to be due to the covert influence of a stronger power over weaker persons, robbing them of their ability to act of their own accord.
- *Mal puesto, hex, rootwork*, and *voodoo death*: Among African Americans and Hispanics, unnatural diseases and death resulting from the power of people who use evil spirits.
- *Nervios* (nerves): In Hispanic cultures, a general state of distress due to life events; it may also be a syndrome that includes "brain aches" or headaches, sleep difficulties, trembling, tingling, *mareos* (dizziness), or simple anxiety and nervousness.
- *Pibalokog*: In Arctic and sub-Arctic Eskimo/Inuit communities, excitement, coma, and convulsive seizures resembling an abrupt dissociative episode, often associated with amnesia, withdrawal, and irrational behaviors.

- *Susto* or *espanto* (fright): In Hispanic cultures, a disorder affecting people of both sexes and all ages; it is believed to result from being deeply frightened by an experience they witnessed, resulting in restlessness, listlessness, diarrhea, vomiting, weight loss, or lack of motivation.
- *Taijin kyofusho*: In Asian communities, guilt about embarrassing others and timidity resulting from the feeling that one's appearance, odor, or facial expressions are offensive to other people.

English as a Second Language

Play therapists need to be aware of the role of language, speech patterns, and communication styles in different cultural communities. The families seen may have significant difficulties in communicating with professionals from the dominant culture. They may not have learned English at all, may know only a few words, or may have learned it as a second language. Cultures speaking languages other than English may have many different dialects and slang, and words may have different meanings across a culture; there may also be differences in accents and vocabulary (Kerl, 1999a, 1999b, 1999c).

Indeed, the language and dialect differences that exist within major cultural groupings can be overwhelming. Saldana (2001) outlines some of the possible variations. Among Asians (including Pacific Islanders), the languages spoken include Chinese, Japanese, Cambodian, Laotian, Filipino, Hawaiian, Hmong, Khmer, Vietnamese, and others; many of these (e.g., Chinese) have large numbers of dialects. Hispanic groups include Puerto Ricans, Cubans, Mexicans, Central Americans (e.g., Salvadorans, Guatemalans, Hondurans, Nicaraguans), and South Americans (Argentineans, Venezuelans, etc.), all speaking their own dialects of Spanish and sometimes other languages or dialects as well. The Mexican province of Oaxaca alone has 23 regional indigenous dialects, not including Spanish. Native Americans consist of more than 500 federally and state-recognized tribes, each with a distinct language, culture, oral history, and tradition.

Children or adults who are not confident in their English ability are likely to be reluctant or limited in their communication with play therapists who speak only English. This difficulty may be even greater during times of emotional stress or with emotionally charged material, with the clients reverting back to their native language. Furthermore, the vocabulary for expressing emotions may be difficult to learn, given the abstract concepts involved (Cochran, 1996). Children who are culturally different from their teachers or schoolmates—and a language difference is a significant cultural difference—experience higher stress. Kalish-Weiss (1989) reports that the most significant cultural barrier is pressure to assimilate into the majority culture. Language barriers and assimilation difficulties can cause a play therapist to assume that a client is functioning abnormally (Casado & Gilbin, 2002).

Play therapy can help reduce linguistically diverse clients' emotional stress and tension, can be effective in helping such children adapt to mainstream U.S. culture and develop English-language skills, and can increase vocabulary for feelings as therapists reflect back the children's play (Cochran, 1996). However, play therapists should not make the mistake of considering release of emotion and stress the main goals of therapy. Not all cultures support the expression of emotions. Play therapists should also be sensitive as to who should be included in the treatment sessions. Some cultures have the eldest maternal or paternal family member speak for a family, instead of the mother or father. As noted earlier, a godparent or grandparent may be more of a caregiver than either parent, and may need to be included in the therapy process.

It is important that all clients be assessed in their primary language, with assessment instruments that have been translated into and standardized in the primary language. Therapists should be aware that the dialects spoken by some clients may have idiomatic terms and slang that do not correspond to those in the translated/standardized measures. In order to avoid creating misunderstanding about the assessment, or feelings of judgment and inadequacy in the clients, play therapists must be sure that the clients understand its purpose, use, and application.

Use of Translators

A common mistake play therapists may make in working with clients whose English is limited or nonexistent is using the children themselves as translators for parents or other relatives, especially if a bilingual therapist or translator is not available. Using a child as a translator reverses family roles and ignores power differences in order to communicate, which dramatically alters the communication and may cause more harm than good (Kerl, 1998). Instead, a family and a play therapist should have an agreed-upon interpreter who will agree to guard the confidentiality of the information given (Ramirez, 1999). Problems with having an interpreter can include a lack of familiarity with psychiatric terms or counseling knowledge, along with distortions or deletions of words and concepts, incorrect translation, inappropriate cultural interpretation, or lack of translatable words or concepts (Saldana, 2001). Ideally, clients with significantly limited English should be referred to a bilingual therapist.

Other pitfalls to avoid include using family friends or relatives to convey information; using secretarial, custodial, or domestic staff to assist in translation; and providing insufficient time for an interpreter and a client to be introduced and achieve basic rapport.

If an interpreter is used, strategies that can help include talking to the client, not the interpreter; using short, simple statements; asking one question at a time; speaking slowly, avoiding jargon, and using plain language; and not raising one's voice. The use of a translator can be expected to double the length of an interview. A therapist should be sure that an interpreter and a client speak the same dialect, and should be sensitive to whether either the client or interpreter appears hesitant or embarrassed to share information (Saldana, 2001).

Personal Space, Eye Contact, and Expression

In mainstream U.S. culture, it is common for people to stand about 3 feet apart during personal conversations. However, in other cultures, it may be more typical to stand as far apart as 4 feet (Japanese) or as close as 2 feet (Middle Easterners), or even to be physically touching during conversation (Native Americans); any of these customs can feel awkward to a play therapist who is not familiar with the cultural norms. Consequently, the play therapist may inadvertently pull away or feel uncomfortable, which can have a negative impact on the therapeutic alliance. The client may feel offended or see the therapist as aloof and cold, while the client may be seen as cool (if standing at a distance) or intrusive, rude, or rowdy (if standing very close to or touching the therapist). All this can happen without either person's ever saying a word. Dialogue is essential for exploring this factor, rather than falling back on stereotypical assumptions or misconceptions.

European Americans also tend to seek and encourage direct eye contact, along with active feedback behaviors (leaning forward, smiling, nodding, etc.). In contrast, people from other cultural backgrounds may show respect or deference by not engaging in eye contact or participating more passively in their body language (Saldana, 2001). Play therapists of European descent should not assume that lack of eye contact indicates lack of interest, guilt, or any other negative point. Furthermore, European Americans tend to expect conversations to go in a linear progression, while members of other cultures (e.g., Native Americans) may find it more natural to go in a circular pattern, allowing the eldest to speak first, and for the entire family. There may be long pauses in contemplation of what should be said, with patience in allowing all to have their say, in their own time. Play therapists who are European Americans may find it harder to tolerate periods of prolonged silence than do others from different cultures, and may try to fill the void (Saldana, 2001). Asian cultures view silence as a sign of respect for elders (Sue & Sue, 1973). Other cultures may find it more natural to have many people speaking at once.

Gesturing and facial expressions can vary considerably across cultural backgrounds as well. Assumptions should not be made that someone is cold or distressed, based on lack of facial expression or gesturing. Various body gestures used in mainstream U.S. culture, such as placing hands on hips, looking down at someone, or holding one's head high, can be misunderstood in another culture as offensive or aggressive. Using hand gestures and beckoning with the index finger are insulting to Koreans and Filipinos/Filipinas. Differing levels of voice volume can also be cultural in nature, and can induce irritability in play therapists who are unaware of this factor and of their own cultural identity and experiences. Middle Easterners (especially when in pain or when someone is dying), Hispanics, and African Americans may be loud and boisterous.

RESEARCH ON FORMS OF PLAY THERAPY FOR MULTICULTURAL POPULATIONS

There is a dearth of research on play therapy with multicultural populations. Most of the few studies to date have used child-centered therapy, filial therapy, Theraplay, and group play therapy. It is incumbent on play therapists to conduct more studies and contribute more articles on the effectiveness of different forms of play therapy with multicultural populations.

Although play is a universal language of children, a play therapist must first observe and understand what a child's cultural play may be communicating, in order for appropriate therapeutic interventions to be designed (Coleman et al., 1993). Multicultural play therapy materials must be included in the play therapy room to help foster children's play and convey culturally based beliefs. Materials that represent children's diverse experiences should be supplied, such as multicultural dolls and plastic animals; culture-specific types of play foods; and paints, crayons, and markers to represent diverse skin tones. A therapist must also be aware of what toys or pictures might be considered bad luck or evil in certain cultures, so as to avoid having them in the therapy room. (See the Appendix to this book for more specific suggestions about materials.)

Play assessments are critical before beginning the treatment process in order to understand how a child and family view play. Some Japanese American children find nonstructured or symbolic play threatening (Nagata, 1998), making it difficult to assess the child's symbolic functioning. The use of drawing and expressive arts techniques might be better used with Japanese American children. Far Eastern children, while able to use symbolic processing, might prefer to use indirect, nonverbal communication, which is culturally taught from an early age (Hinman, 2003). Art materials and attention to nuances in communication would be useful for the play therapist (Hinman, 2003). Hispanic culture, in contrast, views play as a milestone in and of itself (Hinman, 2003). Consequently, difficulties in early childhood may be seen by Hispanic family members as a failure to play as expected (Ramirez, 1998). The play therapist must be sensitive to the cultural view and careful to avoid educating the family regarding the developmental benefits of play behavior (Hinman, 2003). The typical Hispanic American family will desire a problem-focused approach from the play therapist. Thus, the play therapist will need to clearly communicate the different behavioral expectations in the playroom and in parent consultation activities with the child (Hinman, 2003).

The Japanese tradition of passive difference to authority (Nagata, 1998) can easily place the child in a play assessment in a conflicting situation. The play therapist, as authority figure, may be asking the child to engage in a frowned-upon activity (play) by the parent. The child is in the dilemma of risking bringing shame upon the parent by engaging in play or avoiding (thereby disobeying the authority). Consequently, the play assessment and the child's responses may be inaccurately interpreted and invalid (Hinman, 2003). Use of art materials and activities might be better to use in light of the nonverbal communication of emotional issues typical of Japanese American families (Hinman, 2003).

Child-Centered Therapy

"*Cuento* therapy" was developed by Costantino, Malgady, and Rogler (1986) to be sensitive to Hispanic culture. *Cuento* therapy uses culture as both content and context. It is a culturally sensitive modality for Puerto Rican children, using traditional Puerto Rican stories and the cultural values and role definitions that are typical in their themes. *Cuento* therapy mimics traditional storytelling in Puerto Rico and presents popular characters that model functional familial relationships (Vargas & Koss-Chioino, 1992). Their study found that the use of *cuento* therapy resulted in reduced trait anxiety, increased Comprehension scores on the Wechsler Intelligence Scale for Children—Revised, and decreased observer-rated aggression in the treated children, compared with control groups receiving traditional therapy or no intervention at all. The results were stable over a year later.

Filial Therapy

Chinese Families

Chau and Landreth (1997) found filial therapy to be effective with Chinese families in the United States. They offered insight into the fact that Chinese child-rearing practices and values are significantly influenced by strong religious roots in Confucianism: "Parental control, obedience, strict discipline, filial piety, respect for elders, family obligations, maintenance of harmony, and negation of conflict are emphasized in Chinese parenting" (Chau & Landreth, 1997, p. 76). Chinese mental health practitioners have begun to question the impact of such parenting on the children, and have advocated for more affection and warmth in interactions for healthy development (Lau, Lew, Hau, Cheung, & Berndt, 1990). Moreover, the stigma often attached to mental illness makes many Chinese families reluctant to seek out mental health services (Sue & Sue, 1990). Culturally, the Chinese do not speak about or disclose personal problems, as doing so will bring shame on the family (Chau & Landreth, 1997). The family may seek out close friends or utilize physical cures, rather than disclose to an unknown mental health professional.

Chau and Landreth (1997) found that filial therapy allowed parents to be the agents in their children's lives. As filial therapy is not problem-oriented, it avoids the cultural stigma of labeling a child as having a mental health problem. By its nature, filial therapy enhances the relationship between parent and child, which is compatible with Chinese values and culture. The instructor spoke in Cantonese, the language of most of the parents, in training 36 parents from three U.S. cities in a large metropolitan area. Half of the parents were in the control group, and half in the experimental group, but all received filial training by the end of the study. Filial therapy skills were learned through didactic instruction, demonstration, and role playing during 2-hour training sessions, which ran weekly for a total of 10 consecutive weeks. Each parent and child engaged in weekly 30-minute play sessions at home, using a specially supplied toy kit.

Results showed that filial therapy was effective in increasing the empathic parenting behaviors of the Chinese parents. Specifically, there were significant increases in attending to the child, following the child's lead rather than controlling the child's behavior, and commenting on the child's expression of feeling or behavior in an accepting manner. The support and encouragement of the other parents in the group also helped to contribute to a decrease in parental stress, and offered a safe environment for learning and being vulnerable. The parents were able to share not only parenting problems, but marital and family problems.

Yuen, Landreth, and Baggerly (2002) conducted a subsequent filial therapy study with immigrant Chinese families in Vancouver, Canada. Each of the 35 parents who volunteered for this study met the following criteria: being a Chinese immigrant; being able to speak and read Cantonese, Mandarin, or English; and having a child between the ages of 3 and 10 years. A 10-week filial therapy program was conducted with 18 experimental and 17 control families. The families had lived in Canada between 1 and 8 years. Results for the experimental group were significant in reducing the perceived stress related to parenting, reducing the perceived problems related to the children's behavior, and significantly increasing in empathic interactions with and acceptance of the children. The results also demonstrated that the Chinese immigrants were able to learn and incorporate new relationship skills during their interactions in the special play sessions with their children. Parental self-concept improved as well. The authors noted that differences in therapists' and parents' cultural backgrounds make it "imperative that filial therapists be sensitive to the sociocultural world of the parents and cultural themes that emerge in interactions with parents" (p. 82).

Manery (2000) reports on the effective use of dual Theraplay with two Chinese-Canadian kindergarten girls and their parents. This was the first time dual-family Theraplay, as opposed to the typical single-family Theraplay format, was used. The girls were close in age, attended the same school, had similar cultural backgrounds, and had similar presenting problems, which allowed for similar treatment strategies and commentary. Dual treatment also allowed to foster a sense of community and support between the children and families that could continue after therapy. Various cultural issues were discussed as critical to the treatment process. Asians are a very large and diverse group composed of at least 53 different ethnic groups including Chinese, Filipinos, Vietnamese, Japanese, Koreans, Cambodians, Laotians, Indonesians, Thais, Malaysians, and others (Pagani-Tousignant, 1992). In Canada, Chinese-Canadians constitute the overwhelming majority of Asian-Canadians. Asian and other cultures tend to be turned off by the cultural and verbal barriers posed by talk therapies. While Theraplay's emphasis on nonverbal communication may be helpful for some Asian clients, its emphasis on visual and physical contact presented other obstacles (Manery, 2000). Asians "rarely touch in public or in the therapy setting, and direct, prolonged eye contact is considered disrespectful" (Pagani-Tousignant, 1992, p. 9). The fundamental unit in Asian and Chinese culture is the family. The traditional Asian family encourages group loyalty and dependence. Harmony is maintained within the family by extreme sensitivity to the feelings of others. Direct confrontation, disagreement, and criticism are deliberately avoided. Candor is considered impolite, a sign of lack of intelligence or lack of civility (Yee & Hennessy, 1982). Shame is the most common emotional reaction to one's own misbehavior as it reflects badly upon the status of the family and community, and so Asian people learn to act very cautiously. Traditional Chinese parents are quite permissive with their very young children and become much more authoritarian as the children get older. In contrast, Theraplay takes an authoritative approach, enforcing clear standards and encouraging reciprocal communication and mutual recognition of rights.

Presenting problems were the children's extreme shyness and withdrawn behavior in class and not speaking to the teacher or peers for 3 months, in spite of talkativeness at home. Eight weekly sessions with a half-hour Theraplay session was followed by a half-hour adult discussion. Work was conducted in dyads with the therapist and the parents watching and gradually including the parents in the activities. At the end of treatment, progress in both girls was noted, with increased parent–child relationships. A disadvantage of the dual-family Theraplay approach was that the parents may have been initially more guarded with each other, trying to save face by not letting the other know of their specific problems and feeling distressed or ashamed in watching the other child progress faster than their own child.

Korean Families

Lee and Landreth (2003) conducted 10-week filial therapy with 36 immigrant Korean parents in the United States. The 36 parents were divided into experimental and control groups, with their children ranging in age from 2 to 10 years. Results indicated that the experimental group significantly increased their level of empathic interactions with their children and their attitude of acceptance toward their children, while significantly reducing their level of stress related to parenting as compared to parents in the control groups.

Jang (2000) conducted a study of filial therapy in Korea with 32 mothers of children between 3 and 9 years of age, divided into experimental and control groups. The study reported that the culture's pressure for academic and social success had pushed parents to emphasize their children's cognitive development while impairing their ability to form warm and empathic relationships with the children. Consequently, adjustment problems and emotional anxiety were increasing.

The filial model was used over an eight-session, 4-week span of training, with additional 30-minute weekly play sessions at home. Because the mothers indicated that they would not be able to participate for a full 10 weeks, the Landreth (1991) 10-week filial therapy training model was shortened to reduce the likelihood of parents' dropping out. Results yielded significant increases in the experimental group's accepting their children and allowing their children self-direction. In addition, these parents achieved a significantly higher score on involvement in adult–child interaction than the control parent did. Because of their increased involvement in their children's lives, the experimental group also scored significantly higher on empathy in adult–child interaction.

All the mothers reported that they had improved relationships with, and sensitivity to the needs of, their children. Anecdotal results included one parent's reported having an alcohol problem for 2 years and stopping it as a result of being in the filial program. Other mothers reported a new awareness of their children's feelings, and of the negative impact their past high expectations had had on their children. Improved couple communication was reported as a side benefit, with six mothers reporting improvement in spousal communication and relationships. Additional side benefits included improved relationships with in-laws, decreases in parenting stress and children's behavioral problems, and the spontaneous formation of a continuing support group. The author concluded that the success of filial therapy was due to its being not only psychotherapeutic but also educational. The educational aspect of filial therapy helped to reduce the parents' resistance to psychotherapy.

Native American Families

Glover and Landreth (2000) conducted filial therapy with Native American parents on the Flathead Reservation in northwestern Montana. The authors noted the high percentage of high school dropouts, the prevalence and severity of depression and other mental disorders, and the limited availability of services and of Native American therapists on the reservation. Filial therapy was felt to be congruent with traditional Native American values, which include deep respect for individuals, involvement of the extended family, and a liberal child-rearing ideology. The culture also encourages parental teaching by example, as well as showing concern for others' feelings and their expression. The authors noted that "filial therapy supports Native American parents in providing a nonjudgmental, understanding, and accepting environment to foster the positive development of their children" (Glover & Landreth, 2000, p. 60). Filial therapy also supports the traditional Native American value of independence: Children are allowed opportunities to make choices without coercion, as it is believed that making a decision for a child will make the child weak.

The study consisted of 25 parents (or other caregivers) who completed the requirements, with 14 placed in the experimental group and 11 in the control group. The experimental group participated in the 10-week model of filial therapy training (Landreth, 1991), 2 hours weekly, with weekly 30-minute special play sessions at home using a specially designed kit. The materials supplied included "play dough, crayons, paper, blunt scissors, nursing bottle, Native American baby doll, blanket, rubber knife, dart gun, Native American doll house family, toy soldiers, car, Lone Ranger-type mask, Tinkertoys, doctor kit, Band-Aids, play money, rope, transparent tape, bop bag, bowling pins, ball, and a cardboard box to be used as a doll house and container for toys" (Glover & Landreth, 2000, p. 67).

Results showed positive gains for the experimental group in four aspects of perceived acceptance of their children, but only a minimal decrease in overall parent stress. Specifically, the experimental group showed increased skill in communicating acceptance, allowing the children self-direction, and being involved with the children during the special play sessions. The greatest improvement was in allowing the children self-direction: The children in the experimental group demonstrated significantly greater self-directiveness and connectedness with their parents. The authors concluded that filial therapy training was an effective model for enhancing empathic responsiveness in the parents and increasing desirable play behaviors in the children. All the children indicated a higher level of comfort and feeling safe in the play session with the parents.

It was noted, however, that this study was not significantly effective in increasing parental acceptance scores, compared with the scores of other populations assessed on the Porter Parental Acceptance Scale. The authors attributed this to the sporadic attendance of parents at group meetings, which was thought to be due to the cultural priority of family and friends over other obligations, including work, school, or appointments. This study also was not significantly effective in decreasing parental stress scores, compared with the scores of other populations measured by the Parent Stress Index. The authors speculated that this could have been because stress often occurs as a result of conflict with the environment, and such conflict was common on the reservation. Also, the fact that Native Americans take the perspective of living as much as possible in the present, and adapting to rather than resisting change, might have resulted in no significant shifts in stress being seen. A final comment was made about the 30% attrition rate in the filial therapy training, perhaps (as noted above) due to commitments to family matters. The authors suggested that having longer training segments with fewer sessions; providing practice play sessions on site; and creating the atmosphere of a social event by providing food, babysitting/entertainment for the children, and transportation might make the training more attractive. The inclusion of family groups—allowing all the children in a family to participate, along with having a partner, older sibling, or grandparent take part in the training—was suggested as another way to lessen attrition rates.

Group Play Therapy

Using group therapy with culturally diverse child clients requires special care. The therapy needs to be especially sensitive to the reactions, needs, and differences that each individual child brings to the group (Glover, 1999). These differences can be seen as strengths, but may also require some education for the other group members—especially if children from more than one culture are included within a group. Glover (1999) sees client-centered group play therapy as being ideal for working with children from different cultural backgrounds because of its accepting and nonevaluative atmosphere. Opportunities for self-direction are maximized. Reflection of each child's thoughts and feelings allows the child to deal with those feelings, and allows all members of the group to feel free to be who they are.

Multicultural Play Styles

Among the factors that need to be considered in forming a play therapy group for culturally diverse children are differences in children's play styles—especially, again, if a group brings children from more than one culture together. Glover (1999) points out that play styles may vary across cultures. African American children are more sensitive to verbal and nonverbal communications, prefer hands-on experiences, and show persistence in completing a task. They may be louder in verbal interactions than peers, which play therapists from other cultures may need to become accustomed to. Hispanic American children tend to move about more and may take breaks from their play. Asian American children tend to be quiet and to play in a more self-contained mode, rather than to be interactive. They (or their parents) may also give gifts to show appreciation, and the play therapist should graciously accept them.

Native American children are not prevented from making mistakes in play unless results are life-threatening. Children are taught to be aware of nonverbal communications, and to learn by watching. Long pauses and silence during play should be expected, and the play therapist needs to be mindful to speak softly. Native American time perspectives are also different from those of other cultures: Time is viewed as circular, and life is lived in the moment. As a result, lateness and absence may be more common than with other children (Glover, 1999). Therapeutic goals should be short-term and oriented toward the present.

Child-Centered Group Play Therapy for Self-Control

Trostle (1988) studied the effects of child-centered group therapy on self-control in 48 bilingual Puerto Rican children aged 3–6. Twenty-four children each were in the experimental and control groups. The experimental group was divided into six play therapy groups, receiving 40-minute sessions weekly for 10 weeks. The control group received unstructured free play for the same time periods with classmates, using toys similar to those used in the play therapy group. The boys and girls receiving child-centered group play sessions showed significant improvements in self-control, as well as higher-developmental-level fantasy and reality play. The boys were more accepting of others than the girls were in both types of settings. Overall self-confidence and self-esteem increased for the experimental group. Martinez and Valdez (1992), reviewing this study, concluded that child-centered group play was useful for Puerto Rican children as a preventive, remedial, or enrichment tool in facilitating social, representational, and adaptive skills.

Short-Term Group Play Therapy after a Disaster

Shen (2002) investigated the effectiveness of using short-term child-centered group play therapy with Chinese school children in Taiwan who had experienced an earthquake in 1999. Only 65 parents, or the parents of 25% of the targeted student population, agreed to participate. The low number appeared to reflect the traditional Chinese culture's unfamiliarity with research, as well as its reluctance to recognize children's distress and mental health needs. Of the 65 children screened, 30 were identified as at high risk for maladjustment, and were divided into experimental and control groups. The researchers used Mandarin Chinese, the official language of Taiwan, to administer measures. A school counselor with training in child-centered play therapy provided the intervention, through groups of three students apiece, in Mandarin Chinese and in the school's playroom. Each play group received 10 group play therapy sessions lasting 40 minutes each during a 4-week span, with each group meeting two to three times per week.

Results showed the effectiveness of group play therapy intervention with these Chinese students who had experienced a destructive earthquake. Children in the experimental group scored significantly lower on self-reported measures of anxiety and suicide risk after play therapy than did the children in the control group. The child-centered group play therapy helped the children to become less apprehensive when facing environmental stress beyond their control. According to the parents, the children's life adjustment also improved.

The researcher found, however, that school-age Chinese children are not encouraged to play. Anecdotal accounts included this one: "My mom said, 'If you spent your time there just for play, you should not participate in the program any more'"(Shen, 2002, p. 54). Another child dropped out close to the end of the sessions because he was punished for his art grades' dropping. Consequently, it was hard for some of the students to fully enjoy the intervention program, given the strong emphasis on academics over mental health concerns in the culture. The free-play part of the session also presented a dilemma for some older children, especially the boys. The researcher suggested that children aged 10 and younger were more comfortable and enjoyed the free play more than the children aged 11 and over.

An additional difficulty that arose was the lack of instruments designed for Chinese children, which decreases the validity of the study in measuring mental health conditions. Shen (2002) also suggested—given the fact that play is in conflict with traditional Chinese thoughts, although gaining more value in the developing society—that those wishing to engage in play therapy with Chinese children be encouraged to educate teachers and especially parents on the importance of such mental health interventions. Short-term interventions were suggested to help alleviate concerns about lost classroom time and its interference with academic achievement.

In summary, play therapy is an effective treatment modality for children and families that can be used across and within cultures. Play therapists need to be able to provide culturally sensitive services to multicultural clients. We need to improve our cultural sensitivity by increasing our knowledge about the cultures we work with and how they view play and therapy. We need to expand our ability and flexibility in working with the variety of cultural issues that underlie treatment and understand the impact that it has on the formation of their cultural identity. And, finally, given the significant lack of multicultural play therapy research, we need to increase the research conducted with multicultural clients in order to assess the effectiveness of play therapy as a treatment modality and the limitations it poses due to cultural issues.

REFERENCES

Boyd-Franklin, N. (2003). *Black families in therapy: Understanding the African American experience* (2nd ed.). New York: Guilford Press.

Casado, M., & Giblin, J. (2002). Developing a multicultural attitude in the play room. *Association for Play Therapy Newsletter, 21*(4), 13–14.

Chau, I. Y., & Landreth, G. L. (1997). Filial therapy with Chinese parents: Effects on parental empathic interactions, parental acceptance of child and parental stress. *International Journal of Play Therapy, 6*(2), 75–92.

Cochran, J. L. (1996). Using play and art therapy to help culturally diverse students overcome barriers to school success. *School Counselor, 43*(4), 287–299.

Coleman, V. D., Parmer, T., & Barker, S. A. (1993). Play therapy for multicultural populations: Guidelines for mental health professionals. *International Journal of Play Therapy, 2*(1), 62–74.

Costantino, G., Malgady, R. G., & Roler, L. H. (1986). *Cuento* therapy: A culturally sensitive modality for Puerto Rican children. *Journal of Consulting and Clinical Psychology, 54*(5), 639–645.

Falicov, C. J. (1998). *Latino families in therapy: A guide to multicultural practice.* New York: Guilford Press.

Forehand, R., & Kotchick, B. A. (1996). Cultural diversity: A wake-up call for parent training. *Behavior Therapy, 27*, 187–206.

Glover, G. (1999). Multicultural considerations in group play therapy. In D. S. Sweeney & L. E. Homeyer (Eds.), *The handbook of group play therapy* (pp. 278–295). San Francisco: Jossey-Bass.

Glover, G. J., & Landreth, G. L. (2000). Filial therapy with Native Americans on the Flathead Reservation. *International Journal of Play Therapy, 9*(2), 57–80.

Hines, P. M., Garcia-Preto, N., McGoldrick, M., Almedia, R., & Weltman, S. (1992). Intergenerational relationships across cultures. *Families in Society: The Journal of Contemporary Human Services, 73*, 323–338.

Hinman, C. (2003). Multicultural considerations in the delivery of play therapy services. *International Journal of Play Therapy, 12*(2), 107–122.

Huang, L. N. (1998). Southeast Asian refugee children and adolescents. In J. T. Gibbs & L. N. Huang (Eds.), *Children of color: Psychological Interventions with culturally diverse youth* (pp. 33–67). San Francisco: Jossey-Bass.

Jang, M. (2000). Effectiveness of filial therapy for Korean parents. *International Journal of Play Therapy, 9*(2), 21–38.

Kalish-Weiss, B. (1989). *Creative arts therapies in an inner city school.* Los Angeles: Los Angeles Unified School District and Los Angeles County Department of Mental Health. (ERIC Document Reproduction Service No. ED 341 911)

Kerl, S. (1998). Working with diversity. *Association for Play Therapy Newsletter, 17*(4), 1, 3.

Kerl, S. (1999a). Asian identity in the U.S.: Race or ethnicity? *Association for Play Therapy Newsletter, 18*(2), 3, 10.

Kerl, S. (1999b). Multicultural counseling competency in three simple steps. *Association for Play Therapy Newsletter, 18*(1), 2.

Kerl, S. (1999c). Working with African-American populations: Is race important? *Association for Play Therapy Newsletter, 18*(3), 3.

Kerl, S. (2000a). Counselors needed for American Indian populations. *Association for Play Therapy Newsletter, 19*(2), 21.

Kerl, S. (2000b). Diversity 101. *Association for Play Therapy Newsletter, 19*(4), 11.

Kerl, S. (2000c). Theories reflect a more relational sense of self for women and people of color. *Association for Play Therapy Newsletter, 19*(3), 23.

Kerl, S. (2001). Working with African-American children. *Association for Play Therapy Newsletter, 20*(1), 25.

Koss-Chioino, J. D., & Vargas, L. A. (1992). Through the cultural looking glass: A model for understanding culturally responsive psychotherapies. In L. A. Vargas & J. D. Koss-Chioino (Eds.), *Working with culture: Psychotherapeutic interventions with ethnic minority children and adolescents* (pp. 1–22). San Francisco: Jossey-Bass.

Landreth, G. (1991). *Play therapy: The art of the relationship.* Muncie, IN: Accelerated Development.

Lau, S., Lew, W. J., Hau, K. T., Cheung, P. C., & Berndt, T. J. (1990). Relations among perceived parental control, warmth, indulgence, and family harmony of Chinese in Mainland China. *Developmental Psychology, 26*(4), 674–677.

Lee, M.-K., & Landreth, G. L. (2003). Filial therapy with immigrant Korean parents in the United States. *International Journal of Play Therapy, 12*(2), 67–85.

Lewis, A. C., & Hayes, S. (1991). Multiculturalism and the school counseling curriculum. *Journal of Counseling and Development, 70*, 119–125.

Manery, G. (2000). Dual family Theraplay with withdrawn children in a cross-cultural context. In E. Munns (Ed.), *Theraplay: Innovations in attachment-enhancing play therapy* (pp. 151–194). Northvale, NJ: Jason Aronson.

Martinez, K. J., & Valdez, D. M. (1992). Cultural considerations in play therapy with Hispanic children. In L. A. Vargas & J. D. Koss-Chioino (Eds.), *Working with culture* (pp. 85–102). San Francisco: Jossey-Bass.

McGoldrick, M., & Giordano, J. (1996). Overview: Ethnicity and family therapy.

In M. McGoldrick, J. Giordano, & J. K. Pearce (Eds.), *Ethnicity and family therapy* (2nd ed., pp. 1–30). New York: Guilford Press.

Nagata, D. K. (1998). The assessment and treatment of Japanese American children and adolescents. In J. T. Gibbs & L. N. Huang (Eds.), *Children of color: Psychological interventions with culturally diverse youth* (pp. 68–111). San Francisco: Jossey-Bass.

Pagani-Tousignant, C. (1992). *Breaking the rules: Counselling ethnic minorities.* Minneapolis, MN: Johnson Institute.

Ramirez, O. (1998). Mexican American children and adolescents. In J. T. Gibbs & L. N. Huang (Eds.), *Children of color: Psychological interventions with culturally diverse youth* (pp. 215–239). San Francisco: Jossey-Bass.

Ramirez, L. M. (1999. A reader's response to "Working with Latino/a clients: Five common mistakes." *Association for Play Therapy Newsletter, 18*(1), 3–4.

Ritter, K. B., & Chang, C. Y. (2002). Play therapists' self-perceived multicultural competence and adequacy of training. *International Journal of Play Therapy, 11*(1), 103–113.

Saldana, D. (2001). *Cultural competency.* Austin: Hogg Foundation for Mental Health, University of Texas.

Schaefer, C. (1998). Play therapy: Critical issues for the next millennium. *Association for Play Therapy Newsletter, 17*(1), 1–5.

Shen, Y. (2002). Short-term group play therapy with Chinese earthquake victims: Effects on anxiety, depression, and adjustment. *International Journal of Play Therapy, 11*(1), 43–63.

Sue, D. W., & Sue, D. (1973). Understanding Asian-Americans: The neglected minority. *Personnel and Guidance Journal, 12*, 635–644.

Sue, D. W., & Sue, D. (1990). *Counseling the culturally different: Theory and practice* (2nd ed.). New York: Wiley.

Trostle, S. L. (1988). The effects of child-centered group play sessions on social-emotional growth of three-to-six-year-old bilingual Puerto Rican children. *Journal of Research in Childhood Education, 3*(2), 93–106.

Vargas, L. A., & Koss-Chioino, J. D. (Eds.). (1992). *Working with culture: Psychotherapeutic interventions with ethnic minority children and adolescents.* San Francisco: Jossey-Bass.

Webb, N. B. (2001a). Parent–child relationships: A culturally responsive strengths perspective. In N. B. Webb (Ed.), *Culturally diverse parent–child and family relationships: A guide for social workers and other practitioners* (pp. 3–28). New York: Columbia University Press.

Webb, N. B. (2001b). Strains and challenges of culturally diverse practice: A review with suggestions to avoid culturally based impasses. In N. B. Webb (Ed.), *Culturally diverse parent–child and family relationships: A guide for social workers and other practitioners* (pp. 337–350). New York: Columbia University Press.

Yee, B. W. K., & Hennessy, S. T. (1982). Pacific/Asian American families and mental health. In F. U. Munoz & R. Endro (Eds.), *Perspectives on minority group mental health* (pp. 53–70). Washington, DC: University Press of America.

Yuen, T., Landreth, G., & Baggerly, J. (2002). Filial therapy with immigrant Chinese families. *International Journal of Play Therapy, 11*(2), 63–90.

4

❧

The Impact of Culture
on Art Therapy with Children

CATHY A. MALCHIODI

Play therapists, art therapists, psychologists, counselors, social workers, and others often utilize art activities in their work with children. Art therapy—a recognized treatment modality based on the idea that the creative process of art making is inherently healing (American Art Therapy Association, 1996)—is often used with children in a variety of settings, including psychiatric, medical, community, and educational (Malchiodi, 2003). Art making is a slightly different experience from play, because it encourages the creation of a tangible product and helps children visually express and record experiences, perceptions, feelings, and imagination. Art expression may be specifically influenced and defined by cultural values, beliefs, and experiences. Therefore, it is important for therapists using art expression as therapy with children to understand how it may be affected by aspects of culture, in order to provide effective and responsible treatment.

Art therapists have addressed the implications of culture for clinical work with a variety of populations, including children (Dokter, 1998; Golub, 1989; Hiscox-Riley & Calisch, 1998; Hocoy, 2002; Hoshino, 2003; Howard, 1991). Most of these contributions have restated the importance of addressing culture in therapeutic work, mirroring what psychiatry, psychology, and mental health counseling have said about cultural sensitivity. In other words, although relatively little is known about the impact of culture on children's art making, there is a general agreement that any therapy—including art therapy—should address and respect culture as an important component of successful assessment and treatment. However, the types of art activities and approaches that work best in theory and practice within a multicultural framework have not been sufficiently explored and defined. This chapter discusses what is known about using art expression in therapy with children, and describes the overall considerations for therapists in providing "culturally sensitive" art therapy to their child clients.

CULTURE AND CHILDREN'S ART EXPRESSION

The relationship between culture and children's artistic expression helps provide a framework for a comprehensive definition of the concept of "culture." Ethnicity; degree of acculturation (see Figure 4.1); location (rural, urban, or other community); regionalization (e.g., the southern, northern, or western United States; see Figure 4.2); family, extended family, and peers; socioeconomic status (SES); gender; and religious or spiritual affiliations (Coles, 1990; Malchiodi, 1998) all influence the content and style of

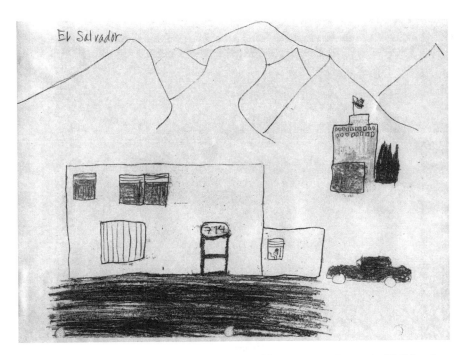

FIGURE 4.1. An 8-year-old boy's drawing of his previous home in El Salvador; the boy and his family had only been living in the United States 3 months and were not yet acculturated to their new home in an urban apartment house.

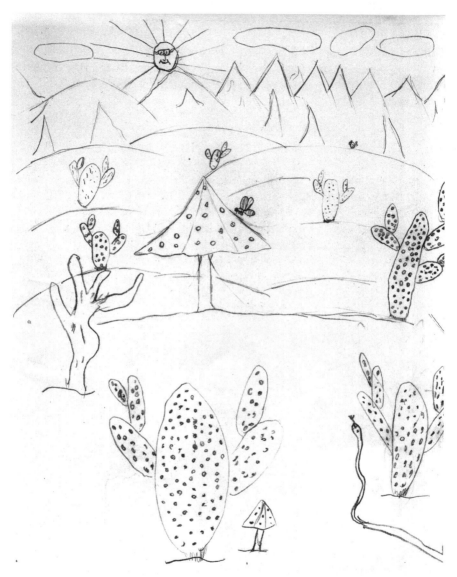

FIGURE 4.2. A 10-year-old girl's drawing of desert scenery from her home in southern Arizona.

children's creative activities. These factors may also affect children's willingness to share and express aspects of the self through drawing or other art activities to varying degrees, depending on how and what is learned through cultural experiences about creative expression.

In addition, the mass media—television, movies, video games, computers, and print material—constitute extremely important element of culture that has a powerful and often direct impact on children's view of themselves (Villani, 2001). Exposure to the media is one of the strongest sources of images, and children adopt images that have had a significant effect on them. The most vivid example in recent years involves the events of September 11, 2001; any child who saw the repeated film footage of the planes hitting the World Trade Center reenacted that image in drawings and play activities for weeks, months, and (in the case of those most severely affected through traumatic loss) years following the attacks. In parts of the United States where films of people falling from the twin towers were televised, children also included falling people in their drawings, in contrast to those children who only saw the planes hitting the buildings (Malchiodi, 2002). In addition to significant events, television, videos, and the World Wide Web are powerful influences on children's adoption of clothing and fashion, as well as on their language, behaviors, and worldviews. These influences are easily recognizable in children's drawings that include references to cartoon characters, popular film or music stars, or movie, television, or video game plots; older children and adolescents may include cultural conventions from peer groups, such as graffiti, gang symbols, or tattoo art (Riley, 1999).

ART EXPRESSIONS OF YOUNG CHILDREN VERSUS OLDER CHILDREN AND ADOLESCENTS

Many therapists who use art activities in their work with children are generally familiar with the normal stages of artistic development proposed by Lowenfeld and Brittain (1987), Gardner (1980), and others that have been used for many decades in evaluation. In brief, these stages include scribbling; basic forms; rudimentary human figures; schematic representations of humans, animals, and objects in the environment; and, eventually, more realistic expressions (for more complete summaries of these stages, please see Malchiodi, 1998; Malchiodi, Kim, & Choi, 2003).

These stages offer a useful guideline in looking at children's drawings—but only up to a point, because they were developed for the most part from observations of children in Western cultures two or more decades ago. In other words, children from diverse ethnic groups and all children from the last two decades (during which time computers have had an increasing impact) have not been thoroughly studied. Despite this lack of contemporary data, the accepted stages of artistic development are generally applicable when one is looking at the drawings of children aged 7 years and younger (Gardner, 1980; Golomb, 1990; Kellogg, 1970). Kellogg (1970) is credited most often for her research on the universal qualities of young children's drawings; she has delineated specific scribbling styles, forms, and constructions of human figures that she believes all normal children experience throughout the world. It appears that at least during the early childhood years, innate factors have a more dominant influence on how children draw and create than cultural ones do.

Golomb (1990) notes that the style and content of art expression is influenced by social factors by age 7 years, when children begin to imitate graphic models in their culture and from a variety of sources, including family, teachers, peers, and the media. From the time that children begin school, they also learn rules for drawing and other types of art expression. For some, these rules involve how to draw specific objects, images, and figures, or even what constitutes a "good drawing" (filling up the entire paper with color or using certain lines or shapes). For example, a child may initially draw a fanciful, imaginative, and colorful bird with a beak and feathers. However, after seeing a simplistic representation of a bird in the form of a "V" in a coloring book or demonstration by a teacher, the child is likely to imitate this symbol for a bird in future drawings, losing many of the earlier qualities (Malchiodi, 1998).

Cattaneo (1994), who has written about art therapy and culture, recalls a childhood memory of her life in Switzerland that illustrates how impressionable children can be when influenced by authorities in their lives:

> I still remember when I was in fourth grade and the knitting teacher brought yarn of different colors for us to choose for knitting a small bag. A girl who lived on one of the poorest streets chose blue and green. The teacher scolded the girl, saying, "Your choice of color really shows where you come from!" This remark strongly influenced my future aesthetics by affecting how I chose certain color combinations. I internalized that blue and green together were "vulgar," and it has taken me a long time to overcome this indoctrinated value judgment. (p. 185)

In many countries, art is a subject expected to be taught by teachers who are recognized and revered as mentors and experts. Quite a few years ago, I was invited to China to train therapists to use art as therapy with children. During my visit, I was asked to work with several groups of 6- and 7-year-olds in schools around Beijing. The children's art expressions were developmentally comparable to children's drawings in the United States (Figure 4.3). However, they were not comfortable with being asked to draw spontaneously, and they requested that I draw a picture for them

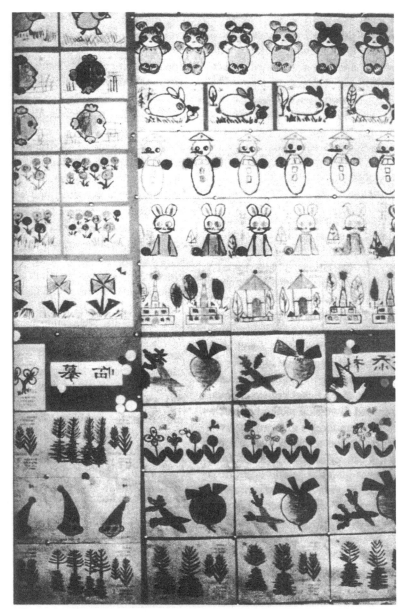

FIGURE 4.3. Drawings by school children, Beijing, China.

to copy. In Asian countries, such as Japan and China, copying the work of an expert is important and is considered a sign of respect to the individual. The children who requested that I provide an example of a drawing for them to reproduce were, in essence, showing me their respect—an important quality within their culture.

Rules about the symbols used in art making can also be culture-specific. For example, in Australian Aboriginal communities, children still learn from elders specific symbols for making human figures (a half-donut shape) and other objects (Cox, 1998). These symbols are traditions handed down for generations whose meanings are recognized by this particular group of individuals—in this case, the Aboriginal community. Children are taught to portray people in a seated position and in a shape commonly accepted within the culture as that which represents "person." In the United States, some Native American children who grow up within tribal communities also learn to draw symbols that are reflective of their culture; if they move from their secluded communities to attend school, they may adopt the drawing conventions of peers, unless the original symbols they learned are reinforced or practiced.

One aspect of children's drawings that is particularly influenced by culture is clothing (Alland, 1983). By the age of 6 or 7 years, most children use some observable visual characteristics to show types of clothing (pants, dresses, shirts, skirts, hats, and footwear), and also begin to differentiate gender through details of clothing. Children in various countries draw images that depict native clothing styles, while those who become acculturated after migration to a new country often adopt the styles prevalent in accepted fashion, particularly those worn by their peers.

ART THERAPY AS A CULTURALLY APPROPRIATE THERAPY WITH CHILDREN

While there are many benefits of art therapy with children (Malchiodi, 2003), several aspects are particularly helpful in work with cultural issues in mind. These include art as nonverbal expression, art as metaphor, and art making as sensory experience.

Art as Nonverbal Expression

Many years ago, I worked as a therapist in a domestic violence shelter for women and their children. My very first child client was a 6-year-old Vietnamese boy, Tao, whose family had recently moved to the United States. Unfortunately, the father was extremely violent to Tao and his mother, forcing her and her children to seek safety and help at the shelter. Tao and I could not verbally communicate with each other; he spoke very little English, and I knew no Vietnamese. However, when he saw a basket of felt marking pens and white paper on the table, he immediately began to draw. His first image was of a large face with eyes, rudimentary nose, and a downturned mouth; the most remarkable features were the large tears he drew in black marker flowing from the face's eyes. He pushed the drawing toward me and whispered something in Vietnamese. I acknowledged his drawing—pointing toward it, making a sad face, and tracing my cheeks where he drew tears on his drawing's face. He nodded affirmatively, and then took his pen and scribbled across the face as if to scratch out the tears; he also drew over the downturned mouth, adding an upturned line over it.

Later in the week, with the help of a bilingual social worker, Tao told me more about his drawing. He said that because he, his younger brother, and his mother had left his father, he was now the "man in the family." Although the face in the picture was originally sad and tearful, Tao felt that he had to be strong for his mother and brother because he was now the oldest male in the family, and stated, "I cannot cry, because I have to take care of my family now." His drawing was a representation of both his sadness and his expected role and responsibilities as the oldest boy in the family.

This experience taught me that when words are impossible due to language barriers, visual expression is a useful form of nonverbal communication. Although a difference in verbal language is one scenario where visual art allows for self-expression, there are other circumstances when a drawing, painting, or clay sculpture can be equally effective. Children may be told or believe that they should not speak about certain events or feelings, but they may be able to express these experiences through art. In some cultures, open expression of emotions is not considered appropriate; in other contexts (especially when abuse or neglect has occurred), children may also learn from parents, other family members, or the community not to talk about specific experiences, or may believe that speaking is not safe or desirable.

Another brief case summary illustrates this point. Tom, an 11-year-old Navajo boy, resided on a reservation with his mother and grandparents. Tom's 16-year-old brother had been in an automobile accident and died from brain and spinal cord injuries. Shortly after his brother's death, Tom's teachers referred him for a psychiatric evaluation because he became extremely agitated and cried often during class. His mother also reported that he had difficulty sleeping; she believed that he was visited by "night spirits," which caused him to scream almost every night.

Tom and his mother left the reservation to seek help through a Native American health center in the nearest large city. After evaluating Tom, the center staff felt that they did not have the services necessary to help him and his mother. They recommended that Tom go to a children's psychiatric unit to receive a more complete evaluation, as well as art and play therapy. After an assessment of Tom's symptoms was made by a child psychiatrist, I saw Tom and his mother for an initial session. Tom spoke openly about his nightmares and his difficulty in staying asleep because, as he said, he feared "ghosts and spirits" were after him. However, after a short while, he felt uncomfortable about saying any more and became quiet and withdrawn.

In brief, there was a taboo among the tribe on speaking openly about deceased persons—in this case, Tom's brother. However, at the suggestion of the Native American health center, Tom was able to draw pictures about his feelings, his traumatic experiences, and eventually even the death of his brother—including what his brother looked like "dead" and the subsequent funeral. During this time, a local medicine man was also consulted and performed a ceremony to aid Tom in his recovery process and to help his mother grieve for the loss of her son. Tom's treatment included both antidepressant medication and art therapy. By the end of 5 months, his depression and anxiety were considerably reduced, and he and his mother returned to their community.

Art as Metaphor

Like play therapy, art therapy offers children the opportunity to use metaphor through nonverbal expression as well as narratives about their creative work (Mills & Crowley, 1986). Ferrara (1994) believes that for certain ethnic populations, art therapy is the therapy of choice when metaphor or symbol is the preferred means of communication. Art can also serve as a metaphor for experiences that a child may feel uncomfortable speaking about because of beliefs or messages from family or community.

Rousseau, Lacroix, Bagilishya, and Heusch (2003) conducted a study with immigrant and refugee children in Canada and observed how art could relay metaphors through image and subsequent storytelling. They asked children to "tell the story of a character of their choice (human or not) who experienced migration in four stages: the past (life in the homeland before migration), the trip itself, the arrival in the host country, and the future" (p. 3). The children drew pictures, and later talked and wrote about each of the drawings. Children who had multiple traumas and losses had difficulties in both drawing the past and projecting themselves into the future. Those who managed to portray images for each of the four stages structured their drawings and stories around three main themes: family, friends, and myths about their home culture.

The researchers concluded from this pilot study and a subsequent study that significant metaphors from a child's culture were helpful in assimilating past experiences with present and future events. They also observed that newly arrived immigrant and refugee children used references to myths and tales from their home culture, their host country, and the cultures of their classmates. When a child predominantly adopted references from the host country, the child might be borrowing a "false self."

One of the strengths of art expression in therapy is its ability to enhance and encourage storytelling and narratives. Stories told about a drawing, painting, or clay sculpture need not be literal to be therapeutic; in fact, a child who has had severe multiple traumas, or who may have serious emotional disorders, may only find it possible to tell imaginative stories about his or her art expressions until trust and the beginnings of attachment are established between therapist and child. The narrative is often a projection of the child's problems and conflicts, as well as coping skills and strengths. By working with the child's projections (a form of metaphor), the therapist not only can assist the child, but also can begin to understand the cultural influences behind the stories told.

Art Making as Sensory Experience

Neuroscience is currently informing the field of mental health about why activities such as drawing are important tools in work with children, particularly those who have experienced trauma (Malchiodi, 2003). Art expression may be especially helpful with traumatized children who experience symptoms of posttraumatic stress disorder (PTSD). For these children, the sensory—tactile and visual—aspects of art making, along with therapeutic intervention, may provide an effective combination in the reduction of PTSD (Steele, 2003). Since many of the children therapists see have had experiences of domestic or societal violence, physical or sexual abuse, loss, immigration, homelessness, or multiple foster care situations, art activities can be an effective tool in the amelioration of trauma because of its ability to contain and express sensory memories of feelings, perceptions, and events.

The same sensory experience of art making often stimulates children to behave in ways that mirror experiences outside the art therapy or play therapy room. Children of any ethnic background who have experienced neglect or poverty often react to art materials with specific behaviors. For example, chronically neglected children may hoard items in the therapy room and may even ask to take supplies with them, just as they may hoard or want to take extra food if offered. In my work in domestic violence shelters, safe houses, and shelters for homeless persons, I learned that even an accidental spill of paint across the table might cause children to reexperience violent incidents that had happened at home when a cereal bowl was dropped on the floor or a glass of milk was tipped over. Children, because of previous verbal or physical punishment, may show the same sort of hypervigilance, fear, and anxiety in a therapy setting that they display in their families, after certain incidents have triggered violent reactions from parents or caretakers (Malchiodi, 1997).

CULTURALLY SENSITIVE ART THERAPY

Hocoy (2002) notes, "Art therapy—like its counterpart talk therapy—when practiced across cultures seems to be at best a cautious enterprise" (p. 144). Although there is still much to learn about how culture influences art therapy with children, there are several aspects that culturally sensitive therapists can take into consideration to exercise their own "cautious enterprise."

First, therapists should view children's art expressions as cultural expressions that reflect a wide range of personal and unique experiences. That is, drawings or other art products cannot be viewed solely as representations of emotions or disorders; nor can they be understood simply through the lens of ethnicity, race, SES, family, gender, peers, or the mass media. In taking a culturally sensitive stance to art therapy, it is more important that therapists view the child's creative work contextually and as being reflective of a variety of aspects of culture.

Second, therapists must be sensitive to how they initiate art expression as therapy with children. For example, for some children, a nondirective approach ("Draw anything you want to") may be threatening and counterproductive to developing trust and establishing a safe, comfortable environment for creative expression. Some children may prefer copying images or tracing to doing something original, particularly if their cultural experiences have dictated this as the preferred way to draw or create. This "art behavior" should be accepted and understood as part of who the children are. Others may find may find craft work more desirable, because it is an art form that is recognized, has been previously experienced, or recalls memories of success or self-esteem.

Although a therapist may focus on a variety of topics in culturally sensitive art therapy with children, some specific directives are helpful. The following are just a few themes that therapists can use to get a sense of children's cultural backgrounds:

1. "Draw a picture of your home." Because "home" may mean anything from an actual house to an apartment, or even a shelter for homeless persons or a street dwelling, it is important to request a drawing of "your home" rather than "your house." Therapists may want to ask children, "What makes it special?" or "What don't you like about it?" Drawings of

"your room," "the shelter," or "your neighborhood" can also help therapists to understand more about the context in which their child clients live. I have often asked children to make me a map of their neighborhood, community, tribal reservation, or apartment complex, in order to help me learn more about their family lives, extended families, and social setting.

2. "Draw a picture of your favorite heroes, or favorite storybook, folktale, or cartoon characters." Along the same line, a therapist may ask a child to draw or create an image from clay of a scene from a favorite story or folktale. Clay figures allow the child or therapist to enact stories or scenarios through movement.

3. "Draw a picture of how birthdays are celebrated in your home or with your family." Children may also be asked to include anything that makes a birthday special, such as certain foods or decorations. This directive generally stimulates memories of family rituals, customs, and values.

It is also important to consider how art-based assessments support culturally sensitive evaluation and subsequent intervention. Some of the traditional projective tasks, such as a drawing of a house, tree, and person, have not been standardized as assessments from a cultural perspective, and the available research is not applicable within a multicultural framework. Others, such as the Silver Drawing Test (SDT; Silver, 2002), have been tested with diverse populations around the world, but have not been evaluated for their cultural appropriateness with non-Western children. The stimulus images in the SDT (a set of cards with images of people, animals, objects, and environmental elements) may not make sense to all children, because of the emphasis on persons of European descent and elements common to Western culture.

Landgarten (1993) proposes that a "magazine photo collage" can be used as a "multicultural" technique for both assessment and treatment. She bases her premise on the idea that magazine images gathered from a variety of sources can provide a wide range of cultural images for a client to use in self-expression. Although magazines may provide a diverse range of images in terms of ethnicity, gender, SES, and values, there is no research proving that this approach is more efficacious as an assessment tool or intervention with individuals from diverse backgrounds. In fact, it may actually reinforce cultural stereotypes, because the print media portray individuals through specific lenses. These images often help to form cultural values and beliefs, particularly with children and adolescents, who are especially susceptible to the messages they deliver about physical appearance, clothing styles, and behaviors.

One newer assessment tool, the Face Stimulus Assessment (FSA; Betts, 2002), has the potential to be more culturally sensitive. It involves a generally recognized image of a blank face (Figure 4.4) and can be used with

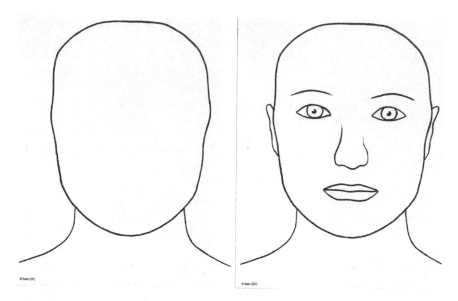

FIGURE 4.4. Face Stimulus Assessment (FSA). From Betts (2002; for more information, please see http://www.art-therapy.us). Copyright 2002 by Donna Betts. Reprinted by permission.

children who do not speak the therapist's language, nonverbal children, or children who are developmentally disabled and have language problems. Figure 4.5 is an example of a completed FSA by an 8-year-old Croatian child whose family members were political refugees and had recently immigrated to the United States. Her drawing of a face, identified as "my mama," also includes the specific type of head wrap and earrings that her mother wore in her native country.

For all of the activities mentioned, therapists should have on hand materials that support and nurture creativity with children of various cultures. For example, there are "multicultural" crayons, felt markers, and clay that come in a range of skin tones approximating skin colors. As previously discussed, photo collage materials should reflect as wide a variety of cross-cultural images as possible, including ethnicities, families, lifestyles, and beliefs. Craft materials such as fabric, yarn, beads, or other objects may be helpful in stimulating some children whose experiences with art have evolved around fabric decoration, jewelry making, or traditional needle arts. The overall caveat is to be aware that children, because of cultural influences, may need a wide range of art and craft materials to inspire and stimulate their creative process in therapy.

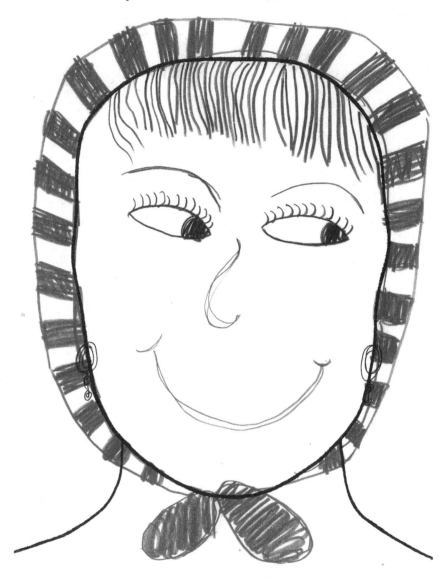

FIGURE 4.5. An 8-year-old Croatian girl's drawing of "my mama."

CONCLUSION

Culture is an important factor in art expression as well as art therapy. Using a comprehensive definition of "culture" in therapeutic work with children—a definition that includes a wide range of social and individual factors—is the foundation of successful art-based assessment and treatment. Art expression allows children to express a variety of life experiences influenced by family, ethnicity, degree of acculturation, SES, beliefs, and numerous other social factors. These experiences are important to decipher and understand before developing any conclusions about children's interests, motivations, psychological status, or creative process. But, most of all, art can offer both children and therapists a form of communication through which to build a healing relationship while simultaneously enhancing and honoring diversity and personal worldviews.

REFERENCES

Alland, A. (1983). *Playing with form: Children draw in six cultures*. New York: Columbia University Press.

American Art Therapy Association. (1996). *Mission statement*. Mundelein, IL: Author.

Betts, D. (2002). *The Face Stimulus Assessment (FSA): Rationale for a new projective drawing test*. Unpublished manuscript.

Cattaneo, M. (1994). Addressing culture and values in the training of art therapists. *Art Therapy: Journal of the American Art Therapy Association, 11*(3), 184–190.

Coles, R. (1990). *The spiritual life of children*. Boston: Houghton Mifflin.

Cox, M. (1998). Drawings of people by Australian Aboriginal children. *Journal of Art and Design Education, 17*(1), 71–79.

Dokter, D. (1998). *Art therapists, refugees, and migrants: Reaching across borders*. London: Jessica Kingsley.

Ferrara, N. (1994). Native American experience of healing through art. *Art Therapy: Journal of the American Art Therapy Association, 11*(3), 216–217.

Gardner, H. (1990). *Artful scribbles*. New York: Basic Books.

Golomb, C. (1990). *The child's creation of a pictorial world*. Berkeley: University of California Press.

Golub, D. (1989). Cross-cultural dimensions of art psychotherapy. In H. Wadeson, J. Durkin, & D. Perach (Eds.), *Advances in art therapy* (pp. 5–42). New York: Wiley.

Hiscox-Riley, A., & Calisch, A. (1998). *Tapestry of cultural issues in art therapy*. London: Jessica Kingsley.

Hocoy, D. (2002). Cross-cultural issues in art therapy. *Art Therapy: Journal of the American Art Therapy Association, 19*(4), 141–145.

Hoshino, J. (2003). Multicultural art therapy with families. In C. Malchiodi (Ed.), *Handbook of art therapy* (pp. 375–385). New York: Guilford Press.

Howard, G. (1991). A narrative approach to thinking, cross-cultural psychology, and psychotherapy. *American Psychologist, 46,* 187–197.

Kellogg, R. (1970). *Analyzing children's art.* Palo Alto, CA: Mayfield.

Landgarten, H. (1993). *Magazine photo collage: A multicultural assessment and treatment technique.* New York: Brunner/Mazel.

Lowenfeld, V., & Brittain, W. (1987). *Creative and mental growth* (7th ed.). New York: Macmillan.

Malchiodi, C. A. (1997). *Breaking the silence: Art therapy with children from violent homes* (2nd ed.). Bristol, PA: Brunner/Mazel.

Malchiodi, C. A. (1998). *Understanding children's drawings.* New York: Guilford Press.

Malchiodi, C. A. (2002). Editorial. *Trauma and Loss: Research and Interventions, 2*(1), 4.

Malchiodi, C. A. (Ed.). (2003). *Handbook of art therapy.* New York: Guilford Press.

Malchiodi, C., Kim, D. Y., & Choi, W. S. (2003). Developmental art therapy. In C. A. Malchiodi (Ed.), *Handbook of art therapy* (pp. 93–105). New York: Guilford Press.

Mills, J. C., & Crowley, R. J. (1986). *Therapeutic metaphors for children and the child within.* New York: Brunner/Mazel.

Riley, S. (1999). *Contemporary art therapy with adolescents.* London: Jessica Kingsley.

Rousseau, C., Lacroix, L., Bagilishya, D., & Heusch, N. (2003). Working with myths: Creative expression workshops for immigrant and refugee children in a school setting. *Art Therapy: Journal of the American Art Therapy Association, 20*(1), 3–10.

Silver, R. (2002). *Art as language.* New York: Brunner-Routledge.

Steele, W. (2003). Using drawing in short-term trauma resolution. In C. A. Malchiodi (Ed.), *Handbook of art therapy* (pp. 139–150). New York: Guilford Press.

Villani, S. (2001). The impact of media on children and adolescents: A 10-year review of research. *Journal of the American Academy of Child and Adolescent Psychiatry, 40*(4), 392–400.

PART II

Play Therapy with Major Cultural Groups

5

❧

Play Therapy in the African American "Village"

SONIA HINDS

There is no Dumpster suitable enough to dump a child.
                    —AFRICAN PROVERB

.

This chapter provides perspectives that will enable the therapist to step into the African American "village" in order to gain insight into the role of play as influenced by slavery, religion, societal factors, socioeconomic status (SES) and gender differences. By gaining this information, the therapist will be better able to form a stronger bond with the "villagers." African American culture-specific data are provided that may be helpful in obtaining a social history. Finally, specific interventions for working with African American children are provided. This author is not aware of any interventions that are used exclusively with African American children; however, some different ways of conceptualizing existing interventions and using the work of noted African Americans in the creative arts are presented here. The resources suggested here for the playroom should not be used to the exclusion of a wide variety of other resources that are commonly used with children of any ethnic group.

One of Virginia Axline's basic principles of working with children is that the therapist should accept the child exactly as he is (Axline, 1969). In order to be fully accepting, a therapist needs to understand a child's culture. To be a true healer to troubled children, it is imperative that the therapist gain cultural understanding by entering the "village" in an attempt to learn the norms, values, and customs—and, where appropriate, weave these into psychotherapeutic interventions.

Although many of the concepts in this chapter apply to most blacks, the term "African Americans" in this chapter refers to the descendents of those who were brought to the United States from the African continent to be used as slaves. References are made to blacks from both inner cities and other areas, and of high, medium, and low SES. The terms "blacks" and "African Americans" are used interchangeably.

The 2001 supplement to the Surgeon General's report on mental health reported that the prevalence of most mental disorders in racial and ethnic minorities in the United States is similar to that of whites, with a few exceptions (U.S. Department of Health and Human Services, 2001). However, it also documented striking inequities in the quality of mental health care of racial and ethnic minorities. One of the barriers deterring these groups from reaching treatment is mistrust of mainstream practitioners (U.S. Department of Health and Human Services, 2001). Mistrust of health care practitioners has deep roots in the African American culture as a result of slavery and its aftermath. Segregation of blacks in schools, health care facilities, and the community during the era of the Jim Crow laws, and continuing (through more covert) discrimination and institutional racism since then, have played a major role in preventing blacks from seeking health care. One major contributing factor to poor care-seeking behaviors is the egregious injustice suffered by African Americans involved in the Tuskegee experiment in the 1930s (Jones, 1993).

Another reason for this lack of trust in health care relates to the over-representation of African Americans in the mental health system; although blacks are reported to have higher rates of schizophrenia and other psychotic disorders compared to whites, the representation in the system even of blacks with these disorders appears disproportionate to that of whites (U.S. Department of Health & Human Services, 2001). A further factor is religious doctrine: Taking one's troubles to another person is seen as unacceptable, because it suggests lack of faith in the power of God. From this point of view, the relationship should not be with the therapist, but with God. In addition, some African Americans may view seeking help from a therapist for children as poor parenting. Finally, older African Americans have taken an oath of secrecy in regard to personal problems. One's "business" is not to be discussed with "people in the street" (Boyd-Franklin, 2003).

In order to raise the quality of care provided to African American children and families, and to foster a trusting client–therapist relationship, it is imperative that cultural competency training be made available to all therapists, including African Americans. One cannot assume that a therapist is culturally competent because he or she happens to be of the same ethnic group as the client. In addition, given the high number of fatherless homes, more male therapists are needed.

To be effective in treating African American clients, therapists of all ethnicities—but especially those of non-African descent—need to understand the African American experience from a cultural and historical perspective. This is begun by understanding racism and its effect on the lives of African Americans throughout generations, and how it trickles down to the child in therapy. A therapist needs to understand what it is to be a black child in America.

RACISM

"Racism" is a belief in the superiority of a particular race, and denial and the use of prejudice based on this belief. Those who hold such a belief view human abilities as being determined by race, and people of other races are treated with antagonism as a result (*Oxford American Dictionary of Current English*, 1999). Many black people, even those who are highly educated, experience racism in some fashion on a daily basis. How this is dealt with is determined by one's upbringing, education, family values, and SES within the black community (Hinkle, 2003).

Beginning in the 1600s (Bennett, 1992), Africans were brought to the Americas from Africa against their will as indentured servants. As slaves, they were denied basic human rights and treated as less than humans. In order to increase the number of slaves available for trade, men and women were forced to procreate with others besides their mates. This led to the practice of having multiple sexual partners. Families were often torn apart as parents or children were sold to different masters; this was the beginning of single parenting and fatherless homes (Bennett, 1992). As of the late 1980s, over half of African American children lived in fatherless homes (U.S. Bureau of the Census, 1990). Slave mothers worked long hours in the fields, leaving their children at home to rear themselves or be looked after by other family members. With this came the start of "kinship bonding" (Gutman, 1976)—the strong family ties and reliance on family members to help raise and protect blood relatives in particular, as well as some who were not blood relatives but considered family. Black males had no control over their families, since a slave owner was the real head of a family. In general, the institution of slavery served to undermine the black family, particularly the role of the black male as competent to support his family (Frazier, 1939). Even though slavery in the United States ended legally in 1863 (with the Emancipation Proclamation) and finally in 1865 (with the end of the Civil War), blacks continued to be subject first to segregation and the Jim Crow laws, and then to less overt but still powerful discrimination and institutionalized racism. They were denied access to good-quality health care, education, decent housing, and job opportunities.

In U.S. society, black males are feared more than females, and they experience racism more intensely. Historically, black males have been kept out of the job market, unable to support their families and fulfill their role in society. This has led to anger, frustration, diminished self-esteem, depression, and other mental health problems (Kunjufu, 1996). Not only have black people had to contend with racism, but some have internalized racial oppression, resulting in self-hatred. This negative self-image has led to "black-on-black" crime; gang activities; domestic violence; drug use; disproportionate involvement in the criminal justice system; and lost generations of strong, gifted, and in many cases highly competent black men. As of the late 1980s, approximately 50% of U.S. federal prison inmates were African Americans (Federal Bureau of Prisons & U.S. Bureau of the Census, 1991). White America has been instrumental in dehumanizing blacks in order to gain control over them and setting blacks against each other since slavery, as exemplified in the infamous Willie Lynch letter of 1712 (Hassan-El, 1999). Blacks have been manipulated into believing that everything "white" is better. Internalized oppression of blacks is seen when blacks glorify white people and their features. Blacks have been so beaten down by racism that some are ashamed of their own culture and even wish they were not black.

My 12-year-old son came home from school one day and related that while practicing for the Christmas play, he noticed that two white children were playing the piano. He asked whether he could play a certain piece and was told "no." The teacher apparently did not believe that he was capable of playing the piano. An African American overheard the conversation and intervened. It was only then that my son was able to play "The Little Drummer Boy" at the Christmas play. Had he not had the support he needed, he could have been left with shame and doubt of his own capabilities.

AFRICAN AMERICAN CHILDREN AND PLAY

Another colleague of this author (M. Kyler, personal communication, 2003) has recalled that during the 1960s, play was the most important part of her day. Play meant freedom from adult supervision and interference. Taking turns being the leader was the norm when children were playing games. Disagreements among friends were solved and did not end in homicide. The neighborhoods were safe, and neighbors looked out for each other's children. Drive-by shootings were unheard of. Children played freely, and they all knew that they had to be home before the street lights came on. Children played hopscotch, double Dutch, and other games, and also created their own games (M. Kyler, personal communication, 2003). Street games such as Sounding the Dirty Dozen, Cans Up, and Ee-Awk-EE were popular (Ariel, 1999).

At the heart of the civil rights movement of the 1960s, there were concentrated efforts to mold and shape the character of black children. After-school programs abounded in storefronts. Although some such programs still exist, today poor neighborhoods are infested with drugs, guns, gangs, and drive-by shootings, which make them unsafe places for children to play. Consequently, these neighborhoods have deteriorated. Organizations such as the Boys and Girls Clubs and the YMCA that do continue to provide organized after-school activities must constantly worry about budget cuts (A. Hinkle, personal communication, 2003).

Black children have few toys that are truly representative of their culture. Toy heroes are for the most part white. When engaging in imaginative play, black children find themselves having to imitate what does not represent them. This communicates to them that "You are not good enough" (Wilson, 1978). Some black girls glorify white dolls with long, silky hair. An African American mother related that her daughter at age 8 was highly upset, because she wanted a white Barbie doll and not a black doll.

A Washington, D.C., school counselor (S. Holt, personal communication, 2003) reported that based on her observation, some African American children in an urban school did not seem to know how to play. Their free developmental play appeared delayed. Upon entering the playroom, they seemed hesitant, cautious, and uncomfortable. This may be attributed to the reality that many of these children are "latchkey" children, and consequently spend too much time watching television and playing video games (S. Holt, personal communication, 2003). However, this view is in direct opposition to that of Ariel (2002), who observed that the free play of low-SES African American children was highly imaginative, with rich sophistication.

African American Parents' Attitudes toward Play

Some African American parents believe that play is appropriate only for young children. They believe that play should stop when the children have developed language skills and when personality and imagination emerge. Such parents' impression is that playing is a stage of development that comes to an end early, and that children need to move on after this. For example, a child may be told that he or she is "too old" to play with dolls or miniature cars. In households where play is understood and provisions for it are made, children are encouraged to engage in various forms of play (S. Holt, personal communication, 2003). Generally, play is influenced by a family's SES. In families where time and transportation are available, children have opportunities to participate in organized sports or after-school activities. However, other parents say that children need more opportunities to engage in free play, rather than spending so much time in these organized activities.

As noted above, children from low-SES homes whose parents are unable to provide for after-school activities may be primarily engaged in talking on the telephone, watching television, or playing video games. In the past, it was not uncommon for parents living in Northern states to send their children to stay with relatives in the South, where they could play freely and bond with family members, during the summer months.

Play as Observed on an Inpatient Psychiatric Child and Adolescent Unit

On a psychiatric ward on which this author worked, it was observed that African American children tended to be very active physically, with lots of moving about and touching. Kunjufu (1995) reflects that some psychologists call this constant movement "verve," which should not be confused with hyperactivity. The play of African American boys was so rough that it bordered on physical aggression, and limits had to be set. What was intended as play or "horsing around" for these children was sometimes misinterpreted as physical aggression by onlookers. However, these young men had a unique way of relating to each other. On the unit, boys' play involved the use of action figures that constantly bumped and crashed into each other, resembling chaos. Miniature cars were pushed around and crashed into each other and into walls. In the sandtray, many figures were placed in the box at one time, with many movements in, around, and under the sand. Strong limits had to be set about the sand in the box. When water was used, there was a great deal of splashing. Rhythmic beats often were created on tabletops with fingers or pencils. Sometimes vocal sounds were made in conjunction to the beats. During group activities, a lot of time was spent trying to get the group members to settle down and ready themselves for the prepared agenda. Latency-age children loved to play with "walkie-talkies" as a way to communicate with each other. Kunjufu suggests that oral tradition is an important component of both black culture in general and black male culture in particular. This is further exemplified by the ability of blacks to excel as rappers.

Card games were played, but an adult was usually present, which helped to keep the children focused. Board games could be tolerated for only a short period, as concentration was lost and the need for body movement was ever-present. Board games that involved "play money" always seemed to have all the pieces together at the end of the game except the "play money." Children loved to stuff their pockets with it, perhaps symbolizing their fantasies of solving financial problems in the home or having their own needs met.

The behavior of the children I observed on the ward can be best understood within a cultural context. African Americans are said to be very spiritual and expressive of their emotions, both physically and vocally. My personal experience is that in most African American church services, the congregation does not sit still. There are hugs, jumping, and shouting and other verbal utterances in response to the sermon and the sense of being moved by the Holy Spirit. It is not uncommon for the preacher to say to the congregation, "Tell the person next to you, 'My God is a good God.'" Through their experience with gospel music and the expression of the Holy Spirit in church, children learn early on to "let it all out" (Cook & Wiley, 2000).

Gender Differences in African American Children's Play

African American male children play with traditional toys designated by our society as toys appropriate for boys, such as army men, cars, wrestling figures, and so on. What was interesting to observe on the psychiatric ward was the attitude of black counselors to the children's play when they perceived that a child was stepping outside the traditional gender role. An 8-year-old client, Robert, carted his toys around by stuffing them in his pockets. When he was given a backpack with pink and lavender trimmings, Robert took the backpack and was rather happy with it. However, a black male counselor openly commented that the backpack for this child was inappropriate because of its "soft colors." Needless to say, the child returned the backpack. On another occasion Robert, who loved to play with dollhouses, could not find the ward's dollhouse. A male counselor who observed how frantic Robert became commented, "Boys don't play with dollhouses." Robert heard the comment and never touched the dollhouse again. This was particularly disturbing, because in the playroom he often used the dollhouse to reenact the abuse he had suffered in his home. The fear among adults of turning males into homosexuals was very strong and sometimes interfered with the children's play. In the black community, homosexuality is much less tolerated than in the white community (Frederick et al., 1991). Because of the history of slavery, a black man's manhood is under constant attack through racism. Adding homosexuality to the black male experience creates another layer of alienation and devaluing. The rough nature of play among black male children could be a fight against what may be perceived as being "gay."

Another factor affecting play among black boys is the "little-man syndrome" (Caviness, 2002). Since about half of African American fathers do not live with their children, a single mother may look to her eldest male child for caretaking responsibilities long before he is ready for these. Often this child has little time for play, because he is seen as a little adult.

Older teenage boys on the ward were also observed engaging in large-muscle activities, such as weight-lifting and arm-wrestling competitions. Watching wrestling competitions on television was prohibited, due to the level of violence, and they protested this bitterly. When they were able to settle down for group activities, there were always several boys in the group with artistic talent who enjoyed drawing and painting. A 13-year-old male who was "stuck" developmentally at a much lower level wanted to be placed in the portion of the unit set aside for younger children, where he would have had more opportunity to play. This child was being raised by three generations of African American women, who allowed him little time to play with peers in the neighborhood, due to the high incidence of crime. Because the clinical staff did not understand his continued need for play and the dynamics surrounding his situation, he was not allowed to be placed with the younger children. Liability issues also did not allow for the flexibility that was needed on the unit.

In the same setting, female African American children aged 8–12 exhibited themes of competition, aggression, anger, rage, and control with the other females. They often competed with their peers for the attention of the males on the unit, who prevented them from working as a group. There were more incidents of physical fights among the girls than there were among the boys, and more incidents of theft involving property such as clothing. There were also more lying and less ability to resolve conflict. Once these issues were worked through individually, the girls were observed having make-believe "tea parties" for each other. Girls were less active and less noisy in their play. They tended to congregate in small groups and seemed to enjoy activities such as coloring, drawing, and playing cards, or activities involving fine motor skills. In sand play, they spent time sifting through, patting, and molding the sand. Girls enjoyed having dolls and stuffed animals on their beds. The older girls enjoyed cooking, preparing meals, and helping with chores. Games such as hand clapping and double Dutch were popular. Girls also enjoyed writing in their journals or diaries. Both males and females enjoyed watching Disney movies.

THERAPIST–CLIENT RACIAL DIFFERENCES: COMMENTS AND SUGGESTIONS

A black client who perceives that a white (or other nonblack) therapist is not down-to-earth, honest, and respectful, or is patronizing, will not be likely to trust the therapist. It is not helpful for clients to hear, "I treat everyone the same," "I don't see color," "Some of my best friends are African Americans," or "You are a credit to your race." Such statements demonstrate lack of racial sensitivity and awareness (Ariel, 1999). In addition, a therapist must understand that not all black people have their roots in Africa, and therefore that there is no "one-size-fits-all" approach. In spite of common bonds, people are uniquely different.

For the most part black people, particularly the older generation, are warm-hearted, but they may expect a therapist to self-disclose before they allow the therapist into their own lives. Self-disclosure remains the choice of the therapist, who should use his or her own judgment (Ariel, 1999; Coustland et al., 1998).

When racial differences exist between a client and therapist, the therapist should invite the client to talk about feelings that could interfere with the therapy process. The client may be uncomfortable or may have preconceived ideas about the therapist. An African American client may request only an African American therapist. Whenever possible, the wishes of the child and family need to be respected. Moreover, when such a request is made, the therapist should find out why and not assume that the reason is obvious; it is important to find out what the past experience has been. It should also be noted that not all African American clients want to be seen by African American therapists. A black client may be worried that a black therapist may be less tolerant than a white therapist, because of fears that a black therapist will perceive the client as having failed to overcome the same racial barriers that the therapist has surmounted. In addition, the black client with a negative internalized racial identity may perceive that the services provided by a black therapist will be inferior, particularly if they are provided in a predominantly white clinical setting.

Every therapist must be aware of his or her own cultural norms and values. In addition, it is imperative that the therapist be aware of common myths and racial stereotypes, as well as the positive attributes, capabilities, and contributions of African Americans throughout the world. Therapists must also be aware of their own possible biases toward African Americans. While in therapy supervision, for example, a white student therapist commented to me on how surprised she was to learn that one of her black clients, a mother of 12 children, had had only one male to father all of her children. Regardless of the circumstances, therapists must always be aware of similar transference and countertransference issues that may be triggered by race and ethnicity.

ASSESSMENT

The therapeutic process begins with the assessment of the client. In addition to a social history, the therapist should obtain information about the client's and family's culture. The following are some areas that should be included.

Major Illness in the Family

Medical problems may shed light on family dynamics that affect a child's behavior in the playroom and have implications for treatment. Common medical conditions among African Americans include type 1 or 2 diabetes mellitus, asthma, depression, high blood pressure, sarcoidosis, sickle cell disease/trait, HIV disease, substance abuse, and cancer. (For a fuller discussion, see Walker & Singleton, 1999).

It is useful to gather information about medication adherence and attitude toward medications. The therapist also needs to be able to help the family look at sources of stress that may influence high blood pressure or other chronic medical conditions, and whether such stress may be related to experiences of racism on the job or in the community. For example, a 10-year-old black male was diagnosed with separation anxiety disorder. His father was diagnosed with diabetes mellitus. While the parents were training the children to administer emergency measures to the father in the event of a hypoglycemic attack, this child became anxious and found it difficult to leave his father's side. Although such a situation could easily have occurred in a white child, this situation was compounded because the child's father was also fighting a racial discrimination case on the job. The son became even more worried about his father.

Values

Some of the common core values and characteristics that have sustained black families include strong kinship bonds, strong religious orientation, adaptability of family roles, respect for elders, and tremendous overall strength and resilience. Denby (2001) provides a more detailed discussion of the resilience of African American families.

A brief discussion of Kwanzaa is appropriate in the context of values. Kwanzaa was created to celebrate the cultural heritage of African Americans; it is not a religious celebration. (Spirituality is discussed separately below.) The seven principles of Kwanzaa—unity, self-determination, responsibility to work together, supporting each other in business, purpose, creativity, and faith—have been adopted as values to live by in some African American families and organizations (Anderson, 1992). There are seven sets of symbols for the celebration: fruits, vegetables, and nuts; a straw place mat; a candleholder, called the *Kinara*; seven candles; an ear of corn; gifts; and a cup of unity. The symbols are used during the celebration to help understand the seven principles or themes of Kwanzaa, and to help remember important events in African American history and teach them to the next generation. The celebration lasts from December 26 through January 1. A different ritual is performed each day, and candles are lit on the *Kinara*.

Following the celebration, African Americans are encouraged to continue to live the seven principles (Anderson, 1992). Not all African Americans are aware of this celebration, however, and many choose not to observe it.

Spirituality

Many African Americans will seek the advice of a minister before, or instead of, going to a therapist for family problems or mental health reasons. Seeking help outside the church may be seen as a contradiction and betrayal of Biblical teachings. My personal experience is that some African American churches believe only in a Bible-based Christian counseling approach, in which searching through and following the Scriptures are used to solve problems. It is believed that problems are solved by surrendering and "leaving it all on the altar," as well as by prayer. Some churches encourage medical attention for serious mental health problems; however, depression is often seen as weakness or lack of faith in God. When psychotropic medications are prescribed, adherence is a huge problem for the same reasons. In such a case, the therapist can help the family see that God's response to the problem may be acceptance of help offered by the clinician. The therapist can also advocate for mental health teaching among leaders in religious communities (Boyd-Franklin, 2003; Cook & Wiley, 2000).

Nonetheless, religion is a strong source of strength and refuge—a "balm" for dealing with daily challenges. Even young children know the important role of spirituality. An 8-year-old African American male who was hospitalized for disruptive behaviors asked that I take him to Sunday school. I was impressed with his request, because he could have easily asked to be taken to an amusement park.

Another important theme that may emerge in therapy and that is influenced by Biblical teaching is "forgiveness" (Stanley, 1987). A child or family member may talk about forgiving a perpetrator of abuse, because this is what God expects. The belief is that if people forgive in the midst of their pain, their healing will begin. However, this concept may be in direct contradiction of the therapist's belief that the perpetrator needs to be punished and not forgiven, or that the perpetrator should confess or admit to the abuse before forgiveness is granted.

Islam is increasingly common among African Americans (Evans, 1996). Ninety percent of all American converts to Islam are African Americans. Muslims are either of the Orthodox faction or of the Nation of Islam. The Nation of Islam believes that Christianity is used to justify racism, and as such considers it a "white man's religion." For both groups of black Muslims, Islam is a way of achieving religious, economic, social, and political ends (Evans, 1996).

Another controversial concept that may surface in therapy is "self-esteem." Some African American churches maintain that promoting "high self-esteem" to the point that it results in self-centeredness, arrogance, and pride contradicts Biblical teachings of humility and esteeming others as more important than oneself. In churches that adhere to a more literal interpretation of the Scriptures, whether in African American or in other cultures, the concept of "high self-esteem" is indicative of the desire of humans to please themselves instead of pleasing God. Humility (lowliness of mind) and denying oneself (by disregarding one's own interest) require choosing to do what God instructs, rather than choosing to do what one wants to do. The belief is that exaltation and promotion come from the Lord (A. Slade, personal communication, 2003). These concepts, if not properly understood and used in the right context, may indirectly contradict the beliefs of the therapist, who may be promoting positive self-regard and a strong sense of self in a child with internalized anger or depression.

Child-Rearing Principles

The therapist should explore the family's child-rearing practices. How does the family discipline the children, and what are the family's rules? What is the general role of grandparents and other extended family members, and what is their involvement with the children in relation to discipline? What is the quality of kinship ties, and what factors are affecting these?

Traditional African American families value respect, particularly for elders; young children are taught to respond to elders with "sir" and "ma'am" at an early age. However, Kunjufu (1995) writes about the growing disrespect of the present generation of African American children, due to societal changes, absent fathers, and deterioriation of the family. Therapists can be instrumental in helping these parents set limits and utilize community resources to reach the children.

Physical/Sexual Abuse

Physical/sexual abuse is not uncommon, and prevalence rates are higher than we know because abuse is not commonly reported. Often children suffer in silence because of shame and guilt. In the African American community, abuse is an important issue, given the high rates of homes with absent fathers, the presence of paramours, and drug and alcohol misuse (Ganns, 1991). Moreover, individuals who have been physically or sexually abused and have not sought treatment tend to pass this type of victimization on to subsequent generations.

Holidays

Therapists should be aware of holidays observed in the African American community (e.g., Kwanzaa, Juneteenth) and respect them. A therapist may choose not to celebrate a particular holiday, but should not expect a client to be present for an appointment on that day. Public and nonpublic mental health establishments should be sensitive to therapists' and clients' wishes to celebrate particular holidays, and refrain from scheduling clients on those days. For example, not all establishments accept the birthday of Martin Luther King, Jr. as a legitimate holiday, even though it is now officially designated as such by the U.S. government.

Conflict

Therapists should determine how families resolve conflict, express anger, and deal with aggression. In particular, they should inquire about whether children are or have been exposed to domestic violence. Also, are weapons kept in the home? If so, are they loaded or unloaded, and are they kept in a safe place?

EXPLAINING PLAY THERAPY TO PARENTS

Parents (or other caregivers) need to be told that ordinarily children do not have the cognitive ability or the language to express themselves as adults until age 11 or 12, and that play is a way for them to express their thoughts and feelings through toys or to "play out" what they are feeling inside. In play therapy, a therapist expresses empathy and reflects to a child what is observed during the process of play. The child then becomes aware of his or her manner of relating to the world. The therapist creates a safe environment in which the child feels free to express him- or herself. It is also a place where the child learns to respond to limits and take responsibility for choices. The parents should be informed that the purpose of therapy is not to "make the child behave" or take over the parents' role.

SPECIFIC INTERVENTIONS
FOR RACIAL/ETHNIC ISSUES

In order to be most effective, a therapist must be able to help any child and family know and understand aspects of their culture and historical beginnings that have contributed to their present situations. Moreover, one of the goals of therapy is to gain a deeper understanding of self. These concepts are particularly important for a black child and family, because racism is part of the black experience.

The therapist needs to be skilled in understanding how the child in play therapy may be experiencing the effects of racial dynamics and how these are manifested in the child's play. Black boys are often the objects of fear; the darker their skin, the greater the fear by whites and even some blacks. Being able to connect with children and understand their pain, even if they don't talk about it, demonstrates understanding and total regard for their struggles.

The following are specific examples of how a therapist might approach racial/ethnic issues in play therapy. A European American psychiatrist working with inner-city African American children (W. Stage, personal communication, 2003) related that in order to be accepted by these children, he needed to demonstrate that he had "power." This was demonstrated by his ability to beat the children at their own game, whether it was a card game or basketball. Once the children perceived that he had power, he gained their respect. The issue of power—an issue that has been passed down through generations as a result of slavery—was a major theme for these black children. Interacting with a white person of power who did not abuse them served as a corrective emotional experience for them and was therapeutic.

Therapists need to be cognizant of the fact that biracial children may be given preferential treatment based on their skin color. Clues may be seen in such a child's play—for instance, if a black doll is mistreated. The issues of these children, and of other children who overidentify with whites, need further exploration. Another example of such overidentification was seen in a 6-year-old girl who refused to remove the hood of her jacket from her head and used the body of the jacket as "long hair" (B. Savoy, personal communication, 2003).

In a somewhat different example, a 7-year-old child was playing with two action figures. He related that one of them was white. He wanted to say that the other figure was black, but had difficulty getting the words out. When the African American therapist asked why he had trouble with the word "black," he said that his mother had told him it was preferable to say "African American." This was a good opportunity to explore the child's feelings about having a black therapist, and to comment on the child's wish to be sensitive to the feelings of the therapist.

When dealing with physically or sexually abused children, the therapist needs to be aware that abuse has two layers for African Americans. Slavery was an abuse of power, exploitation, and dependency that fostered helplessness. Physical or sexual abuse is an issue of power that can also render the child dependent and helpless.

As noted earlier, therapists need to be cognizant of transference and countertransference issues. Blacks may harbor resentment because of racism and may be leery of the intentions of white people. How do they trust a race of people who continue to betray and abuse them? The Rodney King beating is a good example. Black clients may fear that white therapists may have racist attitudes (and, indeed, this fear is sometimes justified). White therapists should not be shocked, respond in fear, or take negative comments personally, but should show empathy and invite such clients to explore the situation. Even a black therapist working with a black family may communicate negative attitudes if the therapist feels that the family members should have been able to overcome their difficulties.

From personal experience of working in a predominantly white establishment, I have found that it is important for therapists not to assume that the best solution to resistance is to match the client with a therapist of the same racial group. European American therapists who are uncomfortable with African American clients may find this an overly easy solution.

WHAT TO HAVE IN THE PLAYROOM

Interventions from a cultural perspective build self-esteem and a sense of self-worth. Therefore, in addition to the standard toys that are generally recommended for the playroom, toys that help black children get in touch with the black experience are recommended.

Dolls with true African American facial features and of various skin tones, rather than just dolls with European features that have been painted dark brown, are important. It is not uncommon for a child to be offended by a black doll whose skin tone is much darker than her own, partly because of the "pretty baby syndrome" (Hassan-El, 1999; A. Hinkle, personal communication, 2003). In our society, as noted earlier, children quickly learn that black is not beautiful and white is pretty and desirable. Black children with white features may be glorified as being "pretty" within the black community (A. Hinkle, personal communication, 2003).

Black dolls with various textures of hair and with hairstyles such as cornrows are useful, as African American children often struggle with the issue of hair. A child may see dolls with long, soft hair that resembles that of white girls, commonly referred to as "good hair," as more desirable than black dolls with hair that may be short and nappy. This child may be in a difficult situation in the home or school, struggling with a poor sense of self. Black dolls with realistic hair and hairstyles will be useful to help the child play out her feelings and work through them in the playroom with the therapist.

Not only should African American dolls have authentic hair and facial features; they should also have various body sizes and figures that are representative of the culture. Dolls that represent various life roles and careers for both males and females should be included as well, in order to expose black children to blacks in various roles and not just in menial jobs. Dolls that represent the extended family and include grandparents should also be available (F. R. Howell, personal communication, 2003).

African American dolls with authentic characteristics are not easy to obtain, but can be found during the Christmas holidays at bazaars held at African American churches. They may also be located at annual doll shows.

Religious symbols—such as figures of a preacher in the pulpit, choir members, congregation members, a miniature Bible, a cross and other religious symbols, and a church building—are useful, particularly for sand play. Symbols used in other religions, such as the Muslim and Jewish faiths, should also be included. In particular, therapists should be aware of how families grieve for losses, learn what rituals are practiced at funerals, and determine to what extent children are allowed to participate. Appropriate materials can be included to help children use in play to recreate related scenarios.

Medical equipment—including an ambulance, helicopter, a doctor's medical bag with equipment, hospital furniture, and the like—should be available, so that children can reenact medical themes and traumatic incidents such as drive-by shootings.

Toy guns, knives, and weapons are items that parents may oppose, due to the high rate of drive-by shootings and murders among young black males. The therapist may get opposition and will need to make a decision. The wishes of the parents should be respected and honored; however, alternative toys (e.g., toy vehicles) should be provided for aggressive play.

Blacks make up about 12.7% of the civilian population of military age (Halbfinger & Holmes, 2003). Children of military personnel may experience fear, abandonment, and other problems that arise with military life and need to be played out. Therefore, *toy soldiers (both male and female) and ammunition* should be part of the playroom equipment.

Board games that stimulate thinking and expression of feelings, such as those by Richard Gardner (1983), should be included. Board games designed to promote expressions of feelings should include scenarios that are real to the black experience. These will need to be created. Such games should challenge the intellect and promote meaningful dialogue. Some families associate card games with gambling and may not appreciate their children playing cards with the therapist or in a group. Similarly, the rolling of dice in certain board games may be viewed as evil.

Clothes for dress-up (including African outfits) that enable the child to imitate adult roles and adults, particularly grandparents and other members of the extended family, are very useful. (Caution should be taken with hats that are not washable, as they can transmit head lice.) *Kente* cloth should also be available for dress-up or for doll play. *Kente* cloth is popular and is symbolic of the ties between blacks in the United States and in West Africa; it is mostly used by males (Sanders, 2000).

Various *craft materials*, such as feathers, buttons, glitter, Popsicle sticks, glue, scissors, blocks, pipe cleaners, uncooked macaroni, and ribbons of different colors, should be included for creating items. In particular, *beads* should be provided for bracelets and necklaces. Those with letters of the alphabet provide the opportunity to create name bracelets. This can be therapeutic, in that it provides another strategy to affirm and strengthen a child's sense of self. Having a discussion of the meaning and origins of names can be very powerful and even more affirming. Amazing stories can emerge about how children got their names and who was responsible for naming them. Black children in general do not seem to get sufficient positive regard, and every opportunity to reinforce self-worth should be encouraged. In certain parts of Africa, wearing beads to adorn the body is very common. The cowrie shell, which represents prosperity and peace, is found on beaches in certain parts of Africa. This shell is commonly used to make African American jewelry, design masks, and is placed on clothing (Sanders, 2000). In the playroom, the child can identify with cowrie shell beads.

Toy animals—particularly those found in the wild in Africa, such as giraffes, zebras, lions, leopards, and elephants—have strong messages from which children can obtain life lessons. It is customary for some African American families to collect elephants, which represent prosperity, financial blessings, strength, and power, as ornaments. These animals may be used in free play or in the sandtray.

In addition to the items listed above, such items as a feeling chart, as well as storybooks and videotapes that portray African American children, should be visible in the playroom.

USE OF CREATIVE ARTS

Music

The therapist needs to know that some of the most important contributions of African Americans are in the form of music. (Indeed, some of the most successful European American musicians have taken either their inspiration or their actual materials from African Americans.) Children who listen to rap or hip-hop music may be encouraged to bring in the lyrics to the music or have an opportunity to play the music during the session. The meaning of the lyrics could be a point of discussion. When music is needed for relaxation, jazz or blues by popular African American artists such as

Ray Charles, Ella Fitzgerald, and Bessie Smith may be very desirable. African drums for drumming and playing tunes to express anger, sadness, and a range of other feelings are very useful. A xylophone has different tones and can spark various energy levels. Children who are difficult to reach, or who have a difficult time engaging in the therapeutic process, may be open to bringing their favorite song to explore the lyrics in a session. In a therapy session, original song lyrics may be written and tape-recorded as a way to express thoughts and feelings.

Art Materials

Materials for drawing and painting with vivid and lively colors, and materials such as clay for making objects, are essential. Many African American children are gifted artists and enjoy various forms of self-expression. It is important to note that Viktor Lowenfeld (Bearden & Henderson, 1993) was responsible for the initiation of art studies at Hampton Institute (now Hampton University) in 1939. Lowenfeld was a psychologist and refugee from Hitler. While in Vienna, he learned through his work with underprivileged clients that art helped to increase self-respect and brought out hidden talents. Lowenfeld was particularly instrumental in encouraging the work of Charles White, Elizabeth Catlett, and John Biggers, noted African American artists. Most significantly, Lowenfeld used African art to help African American students take pride in themselves and their culture.

Creative arts interventions should be strength-based, representing respect, acceptance, and understanding of the child and family. The reader may want to explore Howard Gardner's theory of multiple intelligences (see Armstrong, 2000), which can be used to determine the child's strengths and to implement interventions. Gardner's premise is that there are eight types of intelligence in which individuals can excel. The standard intelligence quotient is only one way in which one can measure abilities. Being able to identify with and capitalize on creative ways to engage the child in the therapeutic process can be very advantageous in moving toward treatment goals.

THEMES AND GOALS OF PLAY THERAPY WITH AFRICAN AMERICAN CHILDREN

Common themes that may emerge in play therapy with African American children are mistrust, anger, rage, loss, abandonment, attachment issues, and hopelessness. These themes, in addition to the presenting problem, have roots embedded in the African American culture. Mistrust has already been discussed. Anger and rage are likewise understandable: Racism, rejection, discrimination, and devaluation by mainstream society, and then being told by a white therapist how to solve your problems, may be infuriating. Multiple losses or abandonments may include absence of a father in the home; absence of one or both parents because of drug problems or incarceration; loss of dignity and respect through racism; loss of grandparents who have provided structure and consistency; and moves in and out of multiple households (and therefore loss of neighborhood friends).

Attachment difficulty is a common theme among African American children whose parents, for one reason or another, are not able to raise them. These children end up in foster care or with elderly grandparents. Because the bonding that should have taken place during the first 3 years of life did not occur, they exhibit attachment problems. Finally, hopelessness can be very severe. As one 8-year-old said to me, "Why should I improve my behavior? I'll probably be dead before age 15. My father, brother, and uncle are in jail, and I'll end up there, too."

In therapy, the goals of the therapist are to provide the following:

- Empathy and affirmation of feelings.
- Acceptance and understanding of the child's struggles.
- Insight into how the child's thoughts and feelings affect behavior.
- Psychoeducation to the parent/caregiver on parenting.

Goals for the child and parent/caregiver include the following:

- Becoming aware of the relationship among thoughts, feelings, and behavior.
- Becoming aware of maladaptive coping skills, and identifying adaptive coping skills.
- Learning to self-soothe and self-nurture.
- Learning to be assertive in order to get needs met.

Identification and expression of feelings deserve particular emphasis here. Among the basic reasons for therapy are to help children get in touch with their thoughts and feelings, and to help them learn how these affect their behaviors. Commonly, the only feelings most children can name are "mad," "glad," and "sad." They cannot name other feelings, and are not aware that it is okay to have more than one feeling. Often they do not know what to do with their feelings. When they are angry, they are often punished, as angry feelings are not acceptable in school or in the home. Or they become anxious when feeling angry, because they may have witnessed and experienced bad things as a result of someone's anger. Children from overly strict homes may be told, "Children are to be seen and not heard." In addition, boys are not allowed to cry in U.S. society in general and African American society in particular. In play therapy, children are helped to identify feelings and given permission to talk about how they feel. Therapists provide feedback in terms of what they observe in the children's play. Once children are able to see how their thoughts and feelings affect their behavior, they may choose to change the way they relate to the world. The following section describes several play-based techniques to assist children in the healing process of play therapy and growth.

DIRECTIVE PLAY THERAPY

In directive play therapy, the therapist determines the intervention for the child or directs the child (or group of children) to participate in a certain activity or intervention. The interventions presented here can be used in individual and group play therapy in both outpatient and inpatient settings.

Ask the Bugs

Ask the Bugs is a projective technique for expressing feelings that I have developed for children aged 8–12. It may be adapted for adolescents aged 13–16.

Background

Coming up with creative ways to help children open up and talk about what is bothering them is a big challenge. As noted previously, African American children learn early that "you don't put your business out in the street." In my work with hospitalized children on a psychiatric ward, frequent responses to requests to talk were "That is none of your business," "I don't want to talk about that," or "That is private information." The underlying premise is that people are weak if they have problems. As I explored the meanings of these statements, I was challenged to come up with inventive, nonthreatening ways to help the children begin talking about their difficulties.

Materials Needed

Various plastic toy insects and insect-like creatures, including an ant, dragonfly, spider, praying mantis, bee, grasshopper, butterfly, fly, or any other insects or similar creatures that seem appropriate, are placed in the middle of the circle.

Procedure

When I use this technique, I gather up to eight children in a circle sitting on the floor. Each child is asked to choose one "bug." After selecting a bug, they think for a moment about what they know about the bug, and share those qualities that they are aware of. They then share with the group a quality of the bug that they can apply to themselves to improve their situation. For example, ants are industrious, orderly, and disciplined. They are also social: They cooperate with one another, work together, and never seem to bump into each other. After all of the children have had an opportunity to share their thoughts, I share with the group the section from Ted Andrews's book *Animal-Speak* (1993) pertaining to what the bug each child has chosen is trying to teach the child. For example, the ant teaches us "how to build, to be an architect in our own lives, how to construct dreams into reality," and "how to work with others for the good of everyone, how to get along." I give a short explanation if the child does not seem to understand. After this has been completed, I then ask each child to share with the group one situation that "bugs" him or her. In this way, the toy bugs provide a safe distance that enables children to talk about worries. I am always amazed at the ease with which the children are able to talk about what is troubling them with this exercise.

Case Example

Eight-year-old Robert, of whom I have spoken earlier, attended group activities on the inpatient psychiatric unit but rarely participated by contributing to the discussions. The day that the Ask the Bugs exercise was introduced to the group, he sat in the circle but was busy playing with his army men. I gently skipped over him, thinking that he was in no way connected to what was occurring in the group. He quickly reminded me that he did not get a turn to select a bug. I apologized and invited him to participate. He selected an ant and proceeded to tell the group that ants kept busy, that they helped each other by passing items around, and that they were good at building things. In reality, Robert was talking about himself.

In response to the question "What bugs you?", Robert, with his head hanging low, said, "The beatings by my mom." I was astounded by his response, as he had never talked about this before. He had been severely abused and consequently placed in foster care. The group was empathetic. He was told that he did not deserve such treatment and that he was a "good person." The group was able to get in touch with his pain and offer support.

When he saw the praying mantis, another child, Mark, who had been diagnosed with attention-deficit/hyperactivity disorder (ADHD), immediately got down on his hands and knees to demonstrate the position taken by this insect. He said that he could learn patience from the praying mantis (which is thought to resemble a person in prayer, but which can also be thought of as a "*preying* mantis," because it has to wait sometimes for hours for its prey to appear). He shared with the group that he watched a television program on nature and animals in the wild where he learned this information, of which neither the group nor I were aware.

Ask the Animals

Ask the Animals, like Ask the Bugs, is a projective technique I have developed for helping children to begin talking about their problems. It is similar to Ask the Bugs, except that toy mammals are used instead of toy insects and the like. It can be used with children aged 8–12, though in the case example below, I used it with adolescents aged 13–16 on the inpatient psychiatric unit.

Materials

Toy animals such as an elephant, horse, gorilla, giraffe, bear, turtle, leopard, zebra, lion, leopard, and whale are good for this exercise. African stores usually carry carved wooden animals imported from Africa that can be used for this exercise. This technique may also be used with any other toy animals with qualities that the children can apply to their own situations.

Case Example

Ramona, a 16-year-old female who was considered one of the most aggressive young women on the unit, selected an elephant during this exercise. When asked why she chose the elephant, she said that it reminded her of herself because of its size (she was overweight). She then said that elephants have good memories. It is also interesting to note that the elephant is the only known animal to have no predators; this girl was known as a "fighter," and the other children stayed away from her. She demonstrated good insight when she was able to state that in the midst of an altercation (which occurred often), she would be able to follow the staff's directions because she (like an elephant using its memory) would remember that the staff had her best interests at heart. This was a big step for her. She was also told that elephants are known for being gentle and protective of their young. This thought served to introduce to her the ideas that building empathy and compassion for others could be the "antidote" for her aggressive, sociopathic, and delinquent behavior. She eventually discontinued her negative behaviors and was able to move back into the community. This technique was useful in helping Ramona to see herself as she related to the world. She was able to choose to change the way she would respond in the future to redirection.

Further Comments

Both the Ask the Animals and Ask the Bugs exercises can also be used to help children self-soothe and self-nurture. They can be told that when they are feeling upset and angry, they can visualize the animals or bugs they have selected and be reminded of the powerful messages that are communicated. Some of the children will want to keep the animals or bugs they have selected; these serve as transitional objects as well.

It is important that the meaning of each symbol to the child who selects it be explored fully. The therapist should not project his or her own meaning or association. It is only after the child has exhausted all his or her ideas that suggestions are made about other possible meanings.

Therapeutic Stories

Therapeutic stories can be used for children of all ages.

Background

An old African tradition, storytelling is an intervention used by parents to pass down tales and family values, soothe children, spend valuable time, stimulate an interest in reading or narratives, and help the children fall asleep. Therapeutic stories serve some of the same purposes, but are different because they contain metaphors that speak to the unconscious. The use of the unconscious mind is based on the therapist-hypnotist Milton Erickson's (Rosen, 1982) premise that people have the power and ability to heal within their unconscious.

Materials

Therapeutic Stories That Teach and Heal (Davis, 1990) contains therapeutic stories that were written for children in Davis's private practice, together with instructions on how and when to select the stories, the meaning of the metaphors, and which features to change in each story in order to adapt it to individual clients. A number of children's books written by African American authors are likewise very useful for addressing various themes in the playroom. A child can also make up his or her own stories or change the ending to suit the child's own situation. Some children have the gift of writing poetry and may enjoy reading works by great African American poets, such as Maya Angelou, Langston Hughes, Nikki Giovanni, Paul Laurence Dunbar, Amiri Baraka, and many others. Also useful in play therapy are stories about influential blacks who overcame adversity, such as Oprah Winfrey and Ben Carson. *Black Books Galore!: Guide to More Great African American Children's Books* (Rand & Parker, 2001) is a wonderful guide for finding Afrocentric children's books by topics.

Procedure

According to Nancy Davis (1990), therapeutic stories are effective because they speak to the unconscious mind—which, unlike the conscious mind, is alert during sleep, is able to hear and remember events, and contains memories from past experiences. Therapeutic stories are short and entertaining, and involve metaphors that match a child's issues. Their messages convey self-love, power, and the ability to heal from emotional pain. The stories are also similar to cognitive therapy, in that they teach new attitudes and beliefs; in the stories, children can see ways out of their dilemmas. It is important not to explain a story to a child, but to have the child talk about what the story means for him or her.

Therapeutic stories can be effective for a number of problems, including ADHD (which often involves difficulty falling asleep), separation anxiety, difficulty with disclosure of abuse, noncompliance with treatment, narcissistic behaviors/low self-esteem, and self-mutilating behaviors. On the inpatient psychiatric unit, they were used to soothe children at bedtime (see below). They are also effective for this purpose at home and in other types of residential treatment facilities. After a story is told during the daytime in an outpatient or inpatient facility, a child may choose to do work in the sandtray as a way of expressing what was stirred up.

Case Examples

Felicia, a 13-year-old African American female, was admitted to the psychiatric unit for intermittent explosive behaviors in the school and community. Her hospitalization was prolonged, as she showed no progress in treatment. During a group play therapy session, the Ask the Animals technique was used. Felicia boldly selected a skunk. Everyone in the group was asked to describe what went into the decision to select a particular animal. Felicia said that she liked the fluffy tail of the skunk, which reminded her of her ponytail. In addition, skunks spray foul scents to keep people away when they are angry. Felicia did much the same with her behavior; she would yell and scream, which created much havoc on the unit.

Following this exercise, a story was written for Felicia, using the skunk as the main character. The story described how the skunk sprayed others due to anger and rage as a primitive defense mechanism. It then presented a more healthy way out of Felicia's dilemma. In the story, the skunk was acting up to get help for her family. Since Felicia's family was already in treatment, she could discontinue acting up and help her family in a different way. After this intervention, Felicia gradually began to calm down and participate in treatment. Before she was discharged, she asked for a copy of the story to take with her.

During her stay on the unit, Felicia needed to communicate her needs in a different way, because the staff could not "get it." The story of the skunk helped her to do that. The metaphors in the story spoke to her unconscious, and she was able to get what she needed in order to move on. Choosing the most effective story for a child communicates true understanding and acceptance of the child.

Further Comments

On the inpatient unit, nursing staff members were assigned to read stories to children (primarily between the ages of 8 and 12) at bedtime. At first the staffers were resistant because they interpreted this intervention, which was intended to help create calm at night and provide special time with the children, as a reward for good behavior (behavior they were not convinced the children had exhibited). Once the rationale was accepted, the stories were read, and the children responded by decreasing their disruptive behaviors at night—perhaps because they were able to internalize self-soothing. The need for sleep medications decreased as well.

Ball Juggle: A Group Play Therapy Game

Ball Juggle is a game that can be used in group therapy for children of all ages, though it needs to be altered slightly for younger children (aged 6–8).

Background

I discovered this game at a conference on conflict resolution many years ago, and I have since adapted it for group play therapy. It is useful for children with poor attention span and poor impulse control, ADHD, problems with taking turns, and problems with being overcontrolling. This game is used to emphasize concentration, staying on task, and delaying immediate gratification.

Materials

At least three balls are needed; ones that are easy to catch are preferable.

Procedure

To play this game, the children are asked to form a circle. The leader throws the first ball across the room to someone in the circle. Each person gets a turn. The last person throws the ball to the leader. This is repeated at least twice. The second time around, the ball is thrown to the same person as before. Then a second ball is added, and then a third ball. The participants must pay attention in order to keep up with the balls, because another ball comes at them when it is least expected. Children especially enjoy this activity, because it allows for body movement, touching, and interaction. Since throwing the balls accurately may be too difficult for children aged 6–8, these younger children could sit on the floor in a circle and roll the balls instead of throwing them.

The therapist can use this exercise as a metaphor: "Many things come at you in life, and it helps to be prepared." Many effective play therapy techniques build social and interpersonal skills, but also have unconscious meaning.

The Big Chair: Assertiveness Training

The Big Chair is an assertiveness training exercise developed for children and adolescents aged 12–16.

Background

Assertiveness skills can be taught through play-based approaches. One method is to use the Big Chair exercise to illustrate the three types of behavioral responses—namely, *aggressive*, *passive*, and *assertive*. The original Big Chair is a Washington, D.C., landmark that was donated to the District by the owners of a popular furniture store. The gigantic chair, which is anchored on the side of a street in the southeast part of the city, is at least 15 feet high and is an impressive sight. Visualizing the size of the Big Chair helps to drive home the messages communicated in the exercise, while also being fun.

Materials

The exercise begins with showing a photograph of the original Big Chair, either on a transparency with an overhead projector or with a slide projector. Either a full-size chair (a large one with study legs) or a toy chair and people from a dollhouse, and a sandtray, are the other materials needed.

Procedure

The history of the original Big Chair and its significance are explained. Simple, one-sentence explanations of what it means to be aggressive, passive, and assertive are given, along with examples. The therapist then utilizes an actual full-size chair to demonstrate each behavioral response by having a child role-play. Alternatively, a toy chair and people from a dollhouse can be used to demonstrate each behavioral response. For the *aggressive* response, the chair is turned upside down, and the child in the role play pretends to smash the chair. The therapist emphasizes that the person has to be pretty angry to get to that point, because the chair is so big. For the *passive* response, the child hides under the chair as if hiding from the outside world and refuses to come out. For the *assertive* response, the child sits on top of the chair. While sitting in the chair, the child's chest should be pushed out, indicating high self-esteem for having chosen assertiveness over the other choices. The child can also be invited to create a scene in the sandtray illustrating the behavioral responses. The therapist explains that every behavioral response (except, in most cases, aggression) has merit in some situations, and that one needs to know when it is appropriate to use them. Children must never be criticized or ridiculed for choices.

Next, the therapist describes a dilemma children are frequently confronted with, and the role-playing child is asked to choose one of the chair's situations (behavioral responses)—either the chair broken or turned upside down; the chair with the child under it; or the chair with the child sitting on it. The therapist then asks the child "to be" or "give voice to" the child in the chosen situation. The therapist then imparts empathy for the child's being in that particular situation, and helps the child to identify the feelings that emerge from being in the situation. Furthermore, the therapist can help the child determine what is needed to move out of the situation if it seems destructive. Children seem to readily understand the concepts of this exercise because they can connect them with the Big Chair in Washington, D.C.

The Story of Ruby Bridges for Anger Management

I have developed an exercise in which a children's book—*The Story of Ruby Bridges*, by the well-known child psychiatrist Robert Coles (1995)—is used to demonstrate effective anger management for children aged 6–12.

Background

Anger and oppositionality are common themes among children who have been victimized. For such children, the goals are to provide exercises and activities that help them unveil their feelings, heighten their awareness of the maladaptive coping skills that result from pent-up anger, and replace these skills with healthy and productive means of coping. *The Story of Ruby Bridges* recounts the experiences of the young girl who integrated the public schools in New Orleans in the 1960s. The storybook is an excellent one to use with children who have difficulty with anger management, and who find it difficult to let go of painful situations and move on.

Materials

A copy of *The Story of Ruby Bridges* (Coles, 1995) is needed. Alternatively, the videotape of the made-for-TV movie based on the book, *Ruby Bridges* (Palcy, 1998), can be used. The therapist should also obtain basic facts on anger and how to manage it for group discussion.

Procedure

The therapist either reads portions of the book or plays parts of the videotape, and then facilitates a discussion. The following summarizes the major events:

Ruby Bridges had to be escorted to school by federal marshals because of hatemongers who were angry that the New Orleans schools were being integrated. After all the white parents removed their children from school, Ruby was the only child in the classroom. One day on her way to school, she turned away from the federal marshals to face the mob who wanted to attack her. When asked by her teacher what she said to the crowd, she replied that she prayed for the crowd.

In therapy with African American children, the therapist should not be surprised if the theme of forgiveness comes up. As noted earlier in this chapter, unconditional forgiveness of offenders is a Biblical belief and an expectation in black churches even for the most traumatic forms of abuse. Ruby's ability to survive her ordeal was due to her spirituality; the support of her parents, her teacher, and the black community; and her relationship with Robert Coles, who provided an opportunity for play in the context of a therapeutic experience.

Safe Place Drawing

Children of all ages—particularly African American children, who may be beaten down by discrimination, racism, or life circumstances—benefit greatly from having a "safe place" to which they can retreat. Oaklander (1978) created safe place drawing as a therapeutic technique.

The child is taken on a journey and asked to visualize a safe place to retreat for peace and relaxation. The child is then told to draw a picture of the safe place. After the picture is completed, the child is asked to share the work. The child gets to choose to speak "for or with" someone or something in the picture.

CHILD-CENTERED PLAY

Child-centered play is based on Carl Rogers's (1951) client-centered approach to therapy, which has been adapted for children by Virginia Axline. Here the child is in charge, and the therapist follows the child's lead, maintaining only those limits that are essential for the child's safety and for compliance with the rules of the therapy setting. Giving an African American child "adult-approved" power and control can be extremely therapeutic. Too often, the child has had to take on parental roles in order to survive, resulting in anxiety and dyscontrol. In the playroom, this child learns to respond to gentle, appropriate limits. In other situations, the child may be overly controlled, and this form of play can be freeing. Children on the psychiatric unit were often amazed that they were given permission "to be in charge." In response to "In here you can say or do almost anything you want," one child said, "But I can't curse, can I?" Just having permission to exercise the option was good enough. He did not feel the need to use profanity. In a playroom, children—particularly those who are told, "Children should be seen and not heard"—can be who they are or want to be without criticism from adults.

Child-centered play provides an opportunity for the therapist to validate the child's view of the world and life experiences, to be fully present with the child, to travel with the child wherever the play experience takes him or her, and to provide empathy. Parents can also be taught to do these things in the home. This intervention is called "filial family therapy" (Guerney, 1980).

When he entered the psychiatric unit's playroom for the first time, Robert, the 8-year-old child described earlier, asked to see the clock. He reached for the clock in an attempt to turn back the time to allow an additional hour. When time was up, he stuffed his pockets with many toys and refused to leave the room, despite empathic statements by the therapist. He eventually had to be carried out of the room. Robert was communicating his insatiable need for this type of play and attention from the therapist, as he did not get it at home. However, children need to know that play alone cannot meet all of their needs. The structure in the playroom eventually helped him to self-regulate, as he was overstimulated.

BEYOND PLAY THERAPY

In situations where there is no progress or the child is very resistant to treatment, a "unity circle" may be created where family members and members of the community who are important in the child's life come together in a therapy session to demonstrate their love and support for the child. Such a show of support and love may be what the child needs to begin making use of the therapeutic process. Each person gathers in a circle around a sandtray with candles, states why he or she is present, offers an affirmation in support of the child, and then lights a candle.

A "libation"—an African tradition enacted during a ceremonial gathering, in which water is poured over a plant or object or directly on the ground to pay homage to the ancestors—may also be performed (Majozo, 1996). A libation signifies the connection of all African people, respecting the dead as well as the unborn. Including a libation as a therapeutic intervention can be a very powerful tool in further demonstrating respect for the child's culture.

Therapists need to be aware of resources beyond play therapy to be able to recommend to parents ways to help their children grow and develop. A recent book, *The Warrior Method* (Winbush, 2001), offers excellent information on how to raise healthy black boys in our society. Some of these techniques may be adapted for girls as well.

CONCLUDING COMMENTS

In order to facilitate the healing process, a therapist who works with African American children and families in play therapy must do the following:

- Understand the black experience from a culturally sensitive and historical perspective. This may be facilitated by visiting black institutions such as churches and museums, and by attending cultural functions.
- Take time to develop trust—which, when once achieved, is like "money in the bank."
- Be careful not to abuse the position of power that comes with being a therapist by overt or covert racism.
- Accept responsibility for the well-being of the child, regardless of the circumstances. For example, black-on-black crime is everybody's problem, not just black people's problem.
- Advocate for the child even if the family has fallen victim to internalized oppression or self-hatred (e.g., the child is ostracized due to dark skin color or hair texture).

- Help the child and family to appreciate role models within the culture and to draw on family strengths.
- Recognize that the themes of hopelessness, mistrust, loss, anger, rage, poor attachment, and abandonment that may emerge in therapy have deep roots embedded in the cultural experience.
- (For a black therapist:) Set appropriate boundaries with parents who may overidentify with the therapist because he or she is black.
- (For a white therapist:) Be ready to respond to the client who says, "You don't know what it is like to be black, because you're white."
- (For a nonblack therapist:) Don't try to imitate the mannerisms of blacks; just be yourself.

Play therapy techniques must be representative of African American culture and must specifically include fine arts and oral traditions, which are two cornerstones of this culture (Kunjufu, 1995). For the African American child and family, play therapy should be a positive learning experience where the child's strengths and culture are celebrated.

REFERENCES

Anderson, D. (1992). *Kwanzaa: An everyday resource and instructional guide*. New York: Gumbs & Thomas.

Andrews, T. (1993). *Animal-speak: The Spiritual and magical powers of creatures great and small*. St. Paul, MN: Llewellyn.

Ariel, S. (1999). *Culturally competent family therapy*. Westport, CT: Praeger.

Ariel, S. (2002). *Children's imaginative play: A visit to wonderland*. Westport, CT: Praeger.

Armstrong, T. (2000). *Multiple intelligences in the classroom* (2nd ed.). Alexandria, VA: Association for Supervision and Curriculum Development.

Axline, V. (1969). *Play therapy* (rev. ed.). New York: Ballantine Books.

Bearden, R., & Henderson, H. (1993). *A history of African-American artists*. New York: Pantheon Books.

Bennett, L. (1992). *Before the Mayflower: A history of black America*. Chicago: Johnson.

Boyd-Franklin, N. (2003). *Black families in therapy: Understanding the African American experience* (2nd ed.). New York: Guilford Press.

Caviness, Y. (2002, November). Single moms, strong sons: Nine guiding principles for raising boys to be men. *Essence*, p. 216.

Clark, K., & Clark, M. (1939). The development of consciousness of self and the emergence of racial identification in Negro pre-school children. *Journal of Social Psychology, 10*, 591–599.

Coles, R. (1995). *The story of Ruby Bridges*. New York: Scholastic.

Cook, D., & Wiley, C. (2000). Psychotherapy with members of African American churches and spiritual traditions. In P. S. Richards & A. E. Bergin (Eds.),

Handbook of psychotherapy and religious diversity. Washington, DC: American Psychological Association.

Coustland, C. L., et al. (1998). Counseling African American men, Part 1, and Part 3. Multicultural and diversity issues: *1*(4), 197–198.

Davis, N. (1990). *Once upon a time: Therapeutic stories that teach and heal.* Oxon Hill, MD: Author.

Denby, R. (2001). Resiliency and the African-American family: A model of family preservation. In S. Logan (Ed.), *The Black family.* Boulder, CO: Westview Press.

Evans, J. (1996). *Why Islam appeals to African Americans* [Online]. Retrieved from http://www.aol.com/gospeladv/gaoct96chtm

Federal Bureau of Prisons & U.S. Bureau of the Census. (1991). *The survey of inmates of Federal correctional facilities study.* Washington, DC: Federal Bureau of Prisons, Office of Research and Evaluations.

Frazier, E. (193). *The Negro family in the United Sates.* Chicago: University of Chicago Press.

Frederick, A., et al. (1991). Condemnation of homosexuality in the black community: A gender specific phenomenon? *Archives of Sexual Behavior, 20*(6), 579–585.

Ganns, J. A. (1991). Sexual abuse: Its impact on the child and the family. In L. N. June (Ed.), *The black family: past, present and future.* Grand Rapids, MI: Zondervan.

Gardner, R. (1983). The talking, feeling, doing game. In C. E. Schaefer & K. O'Connor (Eds.), *Handbook of play therapy.* New York: Wiley.

Guerney, B. (1980). *Filial therapy: A video demonstration tape* [Videotape]. State College, PA: Institute for the Development of Emotional and Life Skills.

Gutman, H. C. (1976). *The black family in slavery and freedom, 1750–1925.* New York: Pantheon Books.

Halbfiner, D., & Holmes, S. S. (2003, March 30). Military mirrors working-class America. *New York Times.*

Hassan-El, K. M. (1999). *The Willie Lynch letter and the making of a slave.* Chicago: Lushena Books.

Hraba, J., & Grant, G. (1970). Black is beautiful: A reexamination of racial preference and identification. *Journal of Personality and Social Psychology, 16,* 398–402.

Jones, J. (1993). *Bad blood: The Tuskegee syphilis experiment.* New York: Free Press.

Kunjufu, J. (1995). *Countering the conspiracy to destroy black boys series.* Chicago: African American Images.

Kunjufu, J. (1996). *Restoring the village, values and commitment: Solutions for the black family.* Chicago: African American Images.

Majozo, E. (1996). *Libation: A literary pilgrimage through the African American soul.* New York: Writers & Readers.

Oaklander, V. (1978). *Windows to our children: A gestalt therapy approach to children and adolescents.* Moab, UT: Real People Press.

Oxford American dictionary of current English. (1999). New York: Oxford University Press.

Palcy, E. (Director). (1998). *Ruby Bridges* [Videotape]. Burbank, CA: Disney Studios.

Rand, D., & Parker, T. (2001). *Black books galore!: Guide to more great African American children's books.* New York: Wiley.

Rogers, C. (1951). *Client-centered therapy: Its current practice, implications and theory.* Boston: Houghton Mifflin.

Rosen, E. (Ed.). (1982). *My voice will go with you: Tales of Milton Erickson, M.D.* New York: Norton.

Sanders, N. (2000). *A kid's guide to African American history: More than 70 activities.* Chicago: University of Chicago Press.

Stanley, C. (1987). *The gift of forgiveness.* Nashville, TN: Nelson.

U.S. Bureau of the Census. (1990). (Current Population Reports, Series P-20, No. 433). Washington, DC: Author.

U.S. Department of Health and Human Services. (2001). *Mental health: Culture, race and ethnicity* (a supplement to *Mental health: A report of the Surgeon General*). Rockville, MD: Author.

Walker, M. A., & Singleton, K. B. (1999). *Natural health for African Americans: the physician's guide.* New York: Warner Books.

Wilson, A. (1978). *The developmental psychology of the black child.* New York: Africana Research Publications.

Winbush, R. A. (2001). *The warrior method: A program for rearing healthy black boys.* New York: Amistad Press.

6

❧

Therapeutic Play
with Hispanic Clients

SILVINA HOPKINS
VIRGINIA HUICI
DIANA BERMUDEZ

.

This chapter discusses the use of therapeutic play in the treatment of sexual abuse with Hispanic families. The scarcity of literature on the topic has been a motivation for us to synthesize and share our clinical experiences. After a concise literature review, we describe the most prevalent therapeutic issues with Hispanics, followed by a case study presentation and a discussion of special considerations with this population. This chapter is not meant to cover all aspects of using therapeutic play with sexually abused Hispanic children and their families. Rather, the purpose is to provide clinicians with a basic understanding of this work, and to trigger the possibility of dialogue in the mental health arena.

The clinical experiences that feed this chapter come from our work at Abused Children's Treatment Services (ACTS), Inova Kellar Center, Fairfax, Virginia. This program provides outpatient therapy to sexually abused children and adolescents, as well as family therapy and support services. The clients receive a combination of expressive therapies (art, play, and sand) and verbal therapy with an integrative theoretical approach. Treatment includes weekly individual sessions with a primary therapist, as well as group and family sessions as needed. After an 8-week semidirective assessment, the therapist articulates treatment goals to be achieved. The average length of treatment is 9 months. The Inova Hospital in Fairfax, local child protective services, and local mental health agencies refer most of the clients.

REVIEW OF THE LITERATURE

The available literature about play therapy specifically with Hispanic clients is scarce and refers exclusively to children. Based on a preliminary literature review, only two articles (Constantino, Malgady, & Rogler, 1986; Trostle, 1988) and one book chapter (Martinez & Valdez, 1992) address the use of play therapy with this population. Despite the growth of literature in the fields of play therapy and therapy with minorities, it appears that since 1992 there have been no publications about Hispanics in play therapy.

In 1986, Costantino and colleagues (1986) proposed "*cuento* therapy" as a culturally sensitive intervention developed to bridge the gap between the Puerto Rican and Anglo cultures. They investigated a sample of 210 high-risk children and their mothers, randomly assigned to receive *cuento* therapy, traditional therapy, or no therapy. The results showed that *cuento* therapy significantly reduced anxiety and aggression, and increased academic comprehension. They emphasized the need to develop further culturally based interventions.

Trostle (1988) measured the effects of child-centered group play sessions on self-control, free-play, and sociometric ratings of 48 Puerto Rican immigrant children. The children who received group play sessions were rated higher than those in the control group. Trostle remarked that play therapy is an important tool for the adaptation of immigrant children faced with a new school and social context. These two studies are important, as they not only explored the effectiveness of play therapy with Hispanic children, but also advocated for serving their unique therapeutic needs.

Perhaps the most extensive writing on this topic is Martinez and Valdez's (1992) book chapter about cultural considerations in play therapy with Hispanic children. The authors explain the use of structured play therapy with Hispanic children, discuss its advantages and weaknesses, describe play materials and techniques used for assessment, and present three case studies. In addition, they propose a "transactional contextual model" of play therapy, which encourages children to explore their issues by acknowledging the multiple cultural contexts that they are immersed in.

Play therapy for abused children has been documented by Grubbs (1994), by Johnston (1997), by Homeyer and Landreth (1998), and perhaps most extensively by Gil (1991, 1994, 1996b). Malchiodi (1997) and Pifalo (2002) have promoted the use of art therapy with traumatized families. All these authors strongly believe in the benefits of using play therapy with minority clients in the treatment of sexual abuse. In addition, play therapy is complemented with verbal and art therapy, since clients naturally drift between different forms of self-expression and healing. For this reason, although this chapter focuses on play therapy, it mentions other creative therapeutic approaches as well.

MOST PREVALENT THERAPEUTIC ISSUES AND NEEDS

Cultural Values Reflected in Therapy

The Hispanic families seen at the ACTS program present a wide range of challenges, from financial constraints to chaotic lifestyles to cultural adaptation problems. In addition, they are undergoing the stress of the usually recent disclosure of a child's abuse—and, if the abuser is being prosecuted, forensic examinations and interviews, as well as current or future court proceedings.

Generally, parents first contact the program in despair, as they perceive the abuse suffered by their children as irreparable. If a child is female, her family's major concern is to find out whether she has been *dañada* (damaged)—in other words, whether she lost her virginity as a consequence of the sexual abuse. If a child is male, the prevalent concern is the possibility of homosexuality. Many Hispanic parents believe that abused boys, particularly when the abuser is also male, lose their masculinity and become homosexuals. This fear on the part of the parents may be related to the strong Hispanic value of *machismo* (male chauvinism), which highly praises masculinity and male dominance (Falicov, 1998). The fact that these children were vulnerable, were unable to stop the abuse, or have hesitated to disclose it exacerbates the parents' fears.

During the intake interview with the parents, it is critical to empathize with their feelings. Many families feel acute guilt and shame about the abuse, even though they usually have had no responsibility for or control over its occurrence. These feelings are linked to the Hispanic value of family privacy—the belief that family problems pertain only to the family and must be solved without external help. This belief is accentuated when it comes to sexual abuse, because sexuality is a very private matter (and sometimes a taboo) in most Latin American countries (Koss-Chioino & Vargas, 1999). Honoring family members' privacy, and empathizing with their feelings of shame and guilt, are essential for building rapport in the therapeutic relationship.

Two situations are common in intake interviews in which both the mother and the father are present: The father either dominates the meeting, or remains silent and apparently disengaged. In the first dynamic, the male in the family (due to prevalence of *machismo* attitudes) controls most events, including what should be reported about the abuse. In the second situation, that of minimal participation, the Hispanic male's evident reluctance to show feelings or discuss personal problems results from his belief that these are not "male matters" and should concern women only. The concept of therapy is traditionally not held in high regard, and it is usually considered an option for women rather than men.

Cooperation and respect for authority are fundamental values in Hispanic culture. Clinicians must understand and carefully handle family structure and hierarchy. Particularly during the assessment period, it is a priority to build a strong therapeutic relationship with the parents of a child before addressing family issues (Falicov, 1998). Based on our experience, the nature of the therapeutic relationship contradicts Hispanic family hierarchy, because it places the therapist—usually a woman—in a position of authority over the father. The therapeutic recommendations of a female therapist may threaten the father's identity as the most powerful figure, and thus his sense of self-respect. As a result, female clinicians frequently face resistance and *machismo* attitudes from Hispanic fathers.

Therapy for a child tends to be well received by a family, as it does not necessarily involve the adults. However, the parents may show resistance when the therapist attempts to make them part of the child's treatment. Even in occasions when only the mother's participation is requested, the father may interfere in order to control the situation. Many times, this obstruction occurs in the form of refusing to drive family members to therapy appointments, when the family owns only one car and the mother does not drive. Furthermore, many Hispanic fathers are doubtful and suspicious of the therapist's role, as a result of lack of information and the stereotype that therapy is only for those who are "mentally ill" or "crazy" (Falicov, 1998).

Usually, such attitudes dissipate as the therapist slowly gains the family's trust. Sometimes gaining trust with Hispanic families requires investing a certain amount of time in chatting about everyday matters not necessarily related to the presenting problem. To mainstream American families, it may appear to be useless or unprofessional to discuss matters not associated with the presenting problem. On the contrary, Hispanic families usually need to connect through simple everyday matters, in order to perceive the therapist as someone reachable, and therefore trustworthy.

Unequal acculturation levels of family members aggravate the disruption of traditional Hispanic family hierarchy (Sluzski, 1979). The acculturation levels of Hispanic children who have come to the ACTS program vary widely: Some children are recent immigrants; others are immigrants who have lived in the United States most of their lives; and still others are children born and raised here with immigrant parents. Regardless of the children's immigration status, they tend to acculturate faster than their parents, due to growing up with the influence of mainstream American culture. Through this process, they abandon some of their culture of origin's values. Their parents, however, may continue to adhere strongly to traditional values, resulting in potential conflicts in family values and expectations. Common sources of disagreement in Hispanic immigrant families are gender roles, parenting styles, family hierarchy and closeness, and work ethics (Falicov, 1998).

We have observed that many Hispanic parents speak only basic English, whereas their children often grow up speaking English as their first language. It is a common phenomenon in immigrant families that the children are asked to translate from Spanish to English and to facilitate interactions with mainstream American culture for their parents. Unfortunately, this gives children a non-normative amount of power that inverts the traditional family hierarchy, creating conflict and power struggles.

Falicov (1998) recommends that a therapist play the role of "cultural intermediary" between unequally acculturated family members. To assist them in resolving cultural conflict, the therapist "helps to clarify similarities, differences, and philosophical and practical implications, and tries to comprehend the underlying assumptions and societal logic behind each cultural system" (p. 81). Furthermore, the therapist encourages negotiation and compromise among family members.

Respect for authority also emerges in interactions with the therapist. Hispanic clients regard professionals involved in sexual abuse cases as all-powerful authority figures, and frequently seem to assent to everything that they suggest. However, their follow-through with recommendations may be compromised by unspoken disagreement. Because mainstream American culture highly values direct and honest expression of ideas, some professionals tend to interpret compliance as passive aggression or lack of assertiveness. Unfortunately, this lack of awareness about minority cultural values can cause many misunderstandings and conflicts that stunt the cooperation needed for therapeutic progress. Professionals should approach Hispanic clients with respect for their values, and should interpret their assenting behavior as politeness rather than agreement.

In therapy with a Hispanic child, it is crucial to engage parents and other caretakers in the child's treatment. Because both the nuclear and the extended family are highly significant in Hispanic culture, relatives have extensive influence on each other. Therefore, a client's ability to improve in therapy is affected by the actions of family members. Sue and Sue (1999) recommend family therapy in working with Hispanics, because changes in an individual client may have profound effects on the entire family.

Fontes, Cruz, and Tabachnick (2001) found preliminary empirical indication that Hispanics tend to believe that sexually abused adolescents are to blame for going along with sexual overtures and accepting bribes from their abusers. In fact, in our ACTS program, we have observed family and community members accusing female clients of provoking or eliciting the abuse. This causes feelings of guilt in abused children that, added to the low self-esteem and depression typically found in such children, slow down recovery. Recruiting the cooperation of family members and raising their awareness about sexual abuse assure that the family will make the necessary changes for healing to happen.

In general, parental support is associated with the adjustment of sexually abused children ("Sexual Abuse Treatment: Status of the Research," 2002). Since parents of sexually abused children experience significant distress, anxiety, and depression, they require emotional support as well as coping skills. In addition, involving parents in the therapeutic process prevents the possibility of defensive behaviors on the part of the parents. Many times these are caused by misunderstandings between therapist and parents, and by the parents' feelings of exclusion from the child's recovery, with a resulting sense of loss of control.

Cultural factors can also contribute to therapeutic improvements. The Hispanic values of family importance, loyalty, and collaboration (Sue & Sue, 1999) facilitate the involvement of families in treatment. Although family members are initially somewhat reluctant to attend family sessions, loyalty to each other motivates their collaboration. Based on our experience, strong religious beliefs and community support are other characteristics that strengthen some of the families, and thus, support recovery.

Use of Time and Pace of Therapeutic Work

It is our belief that the pace of life is generally faster and more intense in mainstream American culture than in Hispanic culture. This cultural aspect may be reflected in therapeutic work with Hispanics in the form of "slow progress." It is important to understand each client's therapeutic pace in the context of his or her culture of origin. In addition, the use of time in therapy varies with culture and gender. Hispanic boys tend to play freely and prefer to be in control of the choice of therapeutic games and activities, particularly during the assessment period. Conversely, Hispanic girls prefer to be guided by the therapist, ask concrete questions, and interact verbally more than boys (Friedrich, 1995).

Race, Personal Value, and Self-Esteem

Racism exists within minority ethnic groups, contrary to the common belief that it occurs only between different racial groups. Hispanic family members tend to value people according to the color of their skin, eyes, and hair. Those children who most closely resemble white non-Hispanic beauty standards receive more acceptance and appreciation, whereas children with browner skin or dark hair and eyes are perceived as less attractive. This phenomenon results both from parental stereotypes and from the influence of mainstream American discrimination against minorities (Ho, 1992). Some of its consequences may include low self-esteem, as well as competition and conflict between siblings with dissimilar physical features.

CASE EXAMPLE

Juan, an 8-year-old Hispanic boy, was referred to the ACTS by the local child protective services agency. Juan had been sexually abused by his babysitter's son. His parents, Mr. and Mrs. Rodriguez, worked full time as a cook and as a receptionist, respectively. Mr. and Mrs. Rodriguez had immigrated to the United States from Central America in adolescence. Juan and his 3-year-old sister were born in the United States. The parents' English and the children's Spanish were modest. Previous to Juan's abuse, Mr. Rodriguez had struggled with alcoholism and domestic violence, which had caused a temporary marital separation. At the time of this referral, he was in recovery.

During the intake interview with one of us (S. T.), Juan's parents were very concerned about their child's well-being; they also expressed their sorrow and anger about being betrayed by the abuser, a trusted person. As was the case with the Rodriguez family, most mothers of abused children tend to react to the abuse with sadness, whereas fathers become furious and wish to take revenge for the harm that the offenders have done to their children. In addition, Mr. Rodriguez was concerned about whether his son would become homosexual as a consequence of the abuse. As stated earlier, Hispanic culture perceives homosexuality as a social problem and generally discriminates against homosexuals. Mr. Rodriguez feared that in the short term, Juan would repeat behaviors learned from the abuse with other children, and that in the long term, this event would lead to adult homosexual behaviors.

The therapist explained to both parents that some children, but not all, repeat sexual behaviors learned from the abuse. She also provided educational information about sexual abuse and related services offered by the ACTS program, the child protective services agency, the court system, and other services—information that is often overwhelming and confusing to Hispanic families. It was also important to explore the parents' understanding and expectations about therapy, and to make the necessary clarifications.

Inquiring about past family history, the therapist learned that Mr. Rodriguez came from a large family in which he had witnessed and experienced physical and emotional abuse throughout childhood. After immigrating to the United States, Mr. Rodriguez had lost contact with the other members of his family. He expressed that he did not wish to see them, as they had caused him much pain. Mrs. Rodriguez's family history was quite different. She belonged to a small family and had happy memories of childhood and her relationship with her parents. She had frequent communication with her mother in Central America and one of her brothers in the United States.

Juan's parents were asked to fill out a Spanish translation of the Child Behavior Checklist (Achenbach, 1991) for assessment purposes. They were very relieved that the assessment questionnaire and registration forms were in Spanish. They had also been pleased to find out during the first telephone contact that the therapist was Hispanic and could speak their native language. Although they spoke modest English, it was evident that they felt more comfortable using their own language. This is common among Hispanic clients, since stressful situations decrease their ability to express themselves clearly in a second language. In general, people can express feelings and thoughts more easily in their first language. In fact, most Hispanic American children whose first language is English prefer to talk about their feelings in English, even when they can also speak Spanish (Gil, 1996a).

Juan was sad and quiet during his first therapy session. He focused on the toy hospital in the therapist's playroom, simulating a car accident. In his play, he rescued an injured boy, using an ambulance and a helicopter. After the doctors saved the boy's life, his mother went to visit him and hugged him. He repeated this play sequence in several of the following sessions. His only verbal interactions were dialogues between the play characters. He rarely spoke directly or made eye contact with the therapist during his first session. Juan was also reluctant to follow directive interventions, such as drawing a self-portrait and doing a kinetic family drawing. He seemed to have a great need for control over the sessions. His parents and schoolteachers reported similar behaviors at home and school.

Before Juan's fourth session, Mrs. Rodriguez telephoned the therapist to tell her that Juan had said he wanted to die after having an argument with his father. His teacher had communicated that he was making similar statements at school. The therapist discussed a safety plan with the mother and held a session with Juan that day. In the session, Juan clearly expressed his desire to die and his intent to commit suicide. The therapist met immediately with the parents to recommend an urgent appointment with a child psychiatrist, in order to assess whether medication would be helpful as a complement to therapeutic treatment.

Despite the parents' difficulty with understanding and accepting this situation, they took Juan to the local children's hospital, where the doctors

recommended hospitalization for a week. He was diagnosed with dys-
thymic disorder and posttraumatic stress disorder (PTSD), and was referred
to a psychiatrist for ongoing medication management. The therapist also
increased her sessions with Juan to twice weekly, and held family and
marital sessions to provide the parents with basic information about childhood depression, PTSD, and appropriate interventions.

Due to the abuse experience, Juan was hypervigilant, fearful, and dis-
trustful of adult males. He suffered from night terrors, nightmares, and
extreme anxiety. Some of Juan's existing personality traits also became
aggravated by the abuse; he developed more aggressive and defiant behaviors, as well as difficulty following instructions and respecting limits.
Juan showed a lack of awareness of his emotions and lack of expression,
as well as difficulty connecting with other people (traits similar to his
father's). Hispanic *machismo* teaches men to hide emotions and to present
a facade of inner strength (Falicov, 1998). The Trauma Symptom Checklist
for Children (Briere, 1995) was very useful in determining which of Juan's
behavioral challenges were consequences of the abuse and which had
existed previously. This is a relatively short questionnaire (with a Spanish
version) that can be filled out by the child's caretaker, or, by children themselves, depending on age.

After the assessment period, the therapist, in collaboration with Juan
and his parents, set the following treatment goals: (1) to ensure Juan's
physical safety at home and increase his feelings of protection; (2) to foster
Juan's ability to identify and express his feelings; (3) to increase his capacity to respect limits and follow instructions from his parents and teachers;
(4) to create new coping skills and to reinforce existing ones; and (5) to help
the family to process feelings and concerns related to the abuse.

In order to foster Juan's ability to connect with and express feelings,
the therapist invited him to watch the video *Sooper Puppy: Once upon a Feeling* (MTI/Film & Video, 1995). After viewing the film, Juan and the therapist discussed Juan's reactions as well as Sooper Puppy's situation, his
feelings, and how he showed them. Another technique often utilized in the
ACTS program consists of asking children to write down feelings that they
feel most of the time. They are then given a square and asked to "choose a
color that best shows each feeling for you." Juan chose red for anger, violet for fear, black for sadness, and orange for happiness. The therapist then
draws a gingerbread figure and asks the child to use the selected colors to
show the parts of the body where the child feels different feelings, and how
much of each feeling he or she feels. This technique was developed by
Eliana Gil, and she calls it Color Your Feelings. She has found this particularly valuable in assessing abused children's perceptions of and feelings
about alleged abusers as compared to other individuals; in this situation,
she asks a child, "Show your feelings when you are with this or that per-

son." Children as young as 4 can utilize this technique effectively. Juan colored the gingerbread figure's thorax in red and violet, and its head and heart in black and orange. He expressed that when he was angry and fearful, his heart would beat fast, and he would have difficulty breathing. When he was either sad or happy, he thought about the things that caused those feelings, and also felt them in his heart.

This technique is very effective with children between 6 and 8 years old and can be modified to fit the clients' needs. For example, with a non-abused child, a life-size body tracing of the child can be used instead of the gingerbread figure. In Juan's case, this variation could have been too intimidating, as he might have been uncomfortable with physical proximity to the therapist. The gingerbread figure drawing allowed child and therapist to address feelings in a playful way that might be less personal.

Following this session, Juan and his parents watched the Spanish version of the *Sooper Puppy* video (Mitchell, 1995) at home, and later discussed it in a family session with the therapist. Although the family members could have watched the video during a session, the therapist chose to have them watch it at home, in order to exemplify the practice of transferring therapeutic activities from the therapy room to everyday home life. This practice helps to ameliorate the stereotype of therapeutic activities as distant from the clients' lives.

After the family members asked questions and made comments about the video in the family session, the therapist introduced a technique called Feeling Balloons (Kaduson & Schaefer, 1997). Each family member draws three balloons. One of them, called the "all kinds of feelings" balloon, is designated for the family members to write down all feelings that are familiar to them. The second and third balloons are for them to list any concerns or problems, as well as their feelings about them. Finally, each person shows his or her feeling balloons to the other participants. Juan and his father were surprised to find that they had similar feelings of anger and sadness about situations from the past. Mr. Rodriguez said that it had been hard for him to express feelings throughout his life. His wife was clearly excited and said that it was the first time her husband had ever spoken openly about himself. She wrote the feelings of hope and fear in her balloons.

The therapist noticed that Juan's parents had difficulty setting clear limits for his behaviors in family sessions. Juan respected limits in individual therapy sessions, whereas he became quite disruptive when his parents were present. When the therapist related her observations to the parents, they acknowledged feeling helpless about Juan's behavioral problems. The therapist recommended that they attend parenting classes at a local human services agency in order to improve their behavioral management techniques. They agreed to sign up; however, only Mrs. Rodriguez followed up with the recommendation.

In individual sessions, the therapist and Juan worked on increasing his ability to respect limits and follow instructions. One of the interventions consisted of asking Juan to create puppets that represented Juan, his parents, and his sister. Therapists can use store-bought puppets for this technique; however, puppets made by the clients represent their feelings and perceptions more accurately. This is particularly important with minority clients, as mainstream puppet makers rarely portray minorities. The therapist then asked Juan to show with the puppets what happened before, during, and after a problem at home. Next, the therapist invited Juan's family members to participate in this process during several family sessions. The conflicts that the family reenacted with puppets reflected Juan's fights with his sister over toys, his reluctance to obey parental decisions, and the parents' inability to handle the situation. With the help of mediation from the therapist, they developed a set of rules for common conflicts, with positive and negative consequences. The family members wrote down the rules in a contract and signed it. The use of mediation and a contract was very successful with the Rodriguez family.

Problem solving with puppets is quite helpful with Hispanic families; indeed, it can be more appropriate than role playing, because the use of puppets as intermediary elements facilitates the expression of feelings and conflicts. Role playing can expose the clients' feelings too much and present a threat. In addition, due to the Hispanic values of respect and submission to authority figures, role playing can be too intimidating and considered "disrespectful." Puppet play can be used as a substitute for, or a step toward, role plays.

In order to further explore cultural differences, the therapist invited Mr. and Mrs. Rodriguez to make a scenario in the sand depicting their lives in their country of origin. Our play therapy offices include a sandbox painted blue on the bottom and sides. Fine sand is placed in this box, and miniatures are available for placing in the sand to create sand scenarios. Clinicians can use this sand therapy nondirectively ("Use as few or as many miniatures as you like, and make anything that comes to mind"), moderately directively ("Use as few or as many miniatures as you like to build a world") and directively ("Use as few or as many miniatures as you like to make a specific scene, such as what your lives were like in your country of origin"). Mr. and Mrs. Rodriguez made a scene from their hometown, using Hispanic miniatures such as a bus loaded with people (*guagua*), fruits, and traditional dishes. Several miniature people represented themselves and their neighbors talking.

Juan and his parents also made a "world" sandtray about their life in the United States, which contained highly symbolic elements. A clock represented the lack of time and the sensation of "living in a rush." A large question mark symbolized their uncertainty and fear about arriving in the

United States. They also placed miniatures for each family member on a bridge and said that it was a symbol for their transition between Central America and the United States. For this type of play, it is crucial to have miniatures that represent accurately the clients' ethnic characteristics and cultural elements (e.g., traditional ways of transportation like the *guagua*; foods like *pupusas*, as well as the more familiar tamales, quesadillas, and tortillas; etc.).

The interventions described above, which were completed in several sessions and homework assignments, had very good results. Juan's parents and teachers reported his improvements. Mr. and Mrs. Rodriguez also became more involved with Juan's school activities. For the first time, Mr. Rodriguez enrolled in an English class, as he realized the need to communicate well in English. These changes that the parents made seemed to have a positive impact on Juan's self-confidence, self-esteem, and school performance.

To address the treatment goal of creating and reinforcing coping skills with Juan, one of the interventions consisted of having Juan paint a T-shirt that he could wear at night, with the help of his parents. The idea was that fostering his feelings of safety at night would improve the quality of his sleep. Juan painted a superhero, and his parents painted an angel that children in their country of origin pray to before going to bed. The three of them talked about bedtime stories and songs that the parents could read and sing to Juan. Many of them were traditional in the parents' home country and were full of fantasy and mythical characters.

In addition, the therapist suggested using a "dream catcher" (a Native American cobweb-like handicraft believed to trap nightmares and to allow only good dreams to roam). Since the family was enthusiastic about the idea, the therapist later gave them a dream catcher for home. Juan hung the dream catcher over his bed and reported not having any more nightmares. This intervention was helpful for Juan, partly because magical thinking is strong in Hispanic culture (Falicov, 1998). In particular, Hispanic populations of low socioeconomic status tend to believe in miraculously healing objects and characters. This way, the therapist drew upon the clients' cultural beliefs to promote treatment goals.

Throughout treatment, the therapist accompanied the family to appointments with the child psychiatrist, both to act as a translator and to provide emotional support. Such action, which might be considered therapist overinvolvement in mainstream American culture, was quite helpful and appropriate with these clients. It helped to appease the parents' anxiety about whether Juan should take antidepressant medication. Based on our experience, a mental health professional should help clients in situations outside the therapy office, especially when a client lacks linguistic or intellectual abilities. The therapist also continued to provide educational information to Juan's parents about childhood depression, therapy, and medications.

In order to help Juan to process feelings and concerns related to the abuse, the therapist once again used video therapy in individual therapy. The video *Break the Silence: Kids against Child Abuse* (Shapiro, 1994) presents testimonies from abused children of various ethnicities, talking about physical and sexual abuse and neglect. After watching it, Juan and the therapist discussed his impressions and feelings about the content. The therapist also invited Juan to make a magazine photo collage about his thoughts and feelings related to the abuse. Juan utilized photos with facial expressions of feelings of fear, confusion, sadness, and anger. The collage is a highly versatile art medium that requires only paper, magazine photos, glue, scissors, and scraps of colored paper for the client to create images that might not be available in books or magazines. We have had the opportunity to observe that unstructured techniques such as this promote creativity and unique personal expression. This consideration is crucial for recent immigrants adapting to mainstream American culture, because it allows them to incorporate elements from their culture of origin that they might not find in the therapy room. In addition, personal artistic creation is an enriching process that generates the sense of belonging immigrants yearn for.

In another session, the therapist asked Juan to create sand scenarios that showed his world before, during, and after his abuse. The goal was to photograph each of the sandtrays and then paste the photos in a book, where Juan could write a narration to accompany the images. In work with traumatized clients, interventions such as this one can help to establish boundaries between the past and the present. That is, the clients can develop a concrete representation of the past as separate from the future, and this may help them "leave the trauma in the past" and not relive it in the present day. The therapist provided Juan with clay and collage materials for him to create any miniatures that were not available in the playroom.

Juan's sand scenario about the time before his abuse showed a Hispanic boy laughing and playing with other children, in a scene full of leafy trees, flowers, and the sun. He explained that before the abuse he was happy and played with other children without fear or worries. The sandtray depicting the period during the abuse had a Hispanic boy crying in front of a yellow monster with many tentacles. He expressed his inability to stop the abuse from happening. In the third sand scenario, representing the time after the abuse, Juan put the monster in a cage and chose a superhero to show how brave and heroic he felt after he reported the abuse to his mother and the abuser went to jail as a result.

The therapist also read with Juan the book *Back on Track* (Wright & Loiselle, 1997), which addresses sexual abuse of boys and is another excellent resource for clinicians. In order to incorporate Mr. and Mrs. Rodriguez, the therapist translated some parts of the book for them to read alone, and then with Juan. One of the chapters specifically addressed fears of homosexuality in abused children—a significant issue for Juan's family. The therapist then met with both parents to discuss their reflections. Mr. Rodriguez said that he now felt less confused and more comfortable with the topic, and had enjoyed reading the book and talking about it with his son. Mrs. Rodriguez communicated having deep respect for her son's strength in defending himself and overcoming the abuse.

Many other efforts were made to involve Mr. and Mrs. Rodriguez in Juan's treatment, including referring the mother to a support group, and both parents to collateral supportive services. The support group was for Hispanic mothers of sexually abused children (two of us, S. T. and V. H., are cotherapists for this group in Spanish). Some of the topics covered in the group were the different types of child abuse, symptoms of sexually abused children, normal sexual development of children and adolescents, family changes as a consequence of the abuse, services involved in a sexual abuse court case, and sex offenders.

For the past 3 years ACTS has offered these groups, which have greatly benefited not only the mothers but also their families. In the majority of sexual abuse cases of Hispanic families referred to ACTS, the abuser is either the stepfather or the biological father. Following the disclosure of the abuse, the offender is typically removed from the home, and the mother is left with complete emotional and financial responsibility for the family. Because the mothers are nonoffending, they usually do not receive any mental health services. Therefore, the need for a support group for mothers is significant.

Mr. and Mrs. Rodriguez also attended eight sessions of collateral support services (with D. B.). To assess the family dynamics, the therapist invited the family to participate in a modified form of a family art procedure called the Family Art Evaluation (Kwiatkowska, 1978), consisting of (1) individual free-theme drawings, (2) individual family portraits (abstract or representational), (3) warm-up individual scribbles, (4) a joint family drawing developed from a scribble, and (5) individual free-theme drawings.

The family interactions during the evaluation were characterized by a desire for improvement and by difficulty with discipline. Most of the drawings were about the family members doing something positive together, and the interactions were cheerful and respectful. However, when Juan became disruptive toward the end, the parents failed to reinforce the limits. In the absence of parental assertiveness, the child became authoritarian. Although Mrs. Rodriguez was shy and passive, she also made insightful remarks about the need for family unity, especially in the couple. Both through his comments and in his drawings, Mr. Rodriguez affirmed his love for the family and his intention to make amends for past mistakes.

Two possible reasons for Mr. and Mrs. Rodriguez's deficient parenting skills were poor education and a frail marital relationship.

Collateral sessions with the parents focused on determining ways to support Juan's recovery; reinforcing basic parenting skills; processing the parents' perceptions of sexual abuse and their fear of homosexuality; creating awareness of cultural differences between Juan and his parents, as well as their cultural adaptation challenges in the United States; and processing their frustration with the psychiatric services that Juan had received.

One of the techniques utilized with Juan for termination of treatment consisted of creating a book of stories whose morals represented insights that Juan had gained in therapy. Juan produced most of the book with the therapist and finished it with his parents at home, in order to reinforce the transition of knowledge from the therapeutic environment to the home. This technique is based on Costantino and colleagues' (1986) work. One of the stories the child wrote was about Lolita, a turtle who lived alone in a remote place because she did not like talking with other turtles. One time, while carrying something heavy, she heard a loud sound and realized that her shell had cracked. She became desperate, as she could not get help, being so far away from the other turtles. After reflecting and fearing for a few hours, she decided to approach them and ask them to take her to the veterinarian. It was a long and painful walk, but she persevered. Lolita healed quickly and decided to move closer to her friends. The moral of the story was the importance of not being isolated and asking for help when one needs it.

SPECIAL CONSIDERATIONS:
THERAPEUTIC APPROACHES,
TECHNIQUES, AND PLAY MATERIALS

As we have mentioned previously, family therapy is one of the most successful therapeutic modalities with Hispanic clients, although there may be obstacles to obtaining family attendance and participation. We have confirmed on numerous occasions that in work with a child, involvement of the family in treatment is pivotal to progress. Most Hispanic clients with low education lack basic knowledge about psychology and the purpose of therapy. Therefore, it is necessary to explore with Hispanic families their understanding and expectations of therapy, and to clarify any misconceptions that they might have.

Play therapy is particularly valuable with Hispanic families. Due to the stigma of mental illness and therapy, many family members (most frequently men) are initially reluctant to participate in treatment. Nevertheless, they are attracted to interventions based on play, as these bring

together the therapeutic and the day-to-day realms. Playfulness is an inherent human characteristic that allows for freedom and creativity.

Group work is another valuable therapeutic resource, especially for
children who find it difficult and unproductive to express themselves in
individual sessions. Hispanic girls generally enjoy and benefit from group
therapy, as they feel supported by meeting other girls who have experienced sexual abuse. However, some Hispanic boys tend to feel embarrassed
by sharing experiences of this nature with a group; this reaction is consistent with those of boys from other cultures (Friedrich, 1995). Groups for
Hispanic parents are culturally very appropriate, because they reinforce
the existing cultural sense of community and *familismo*. However, the reluctance to talk to strangers has to be overcome. Groups for Hispanic
mothers have tended to develop into familial structures; for example,
members often share a home-cooked meal to celebrate the group's ending.

It is extremely important for therapists to be familiar with culturally
sensitive mental health services in their geographic area, in order to refer
their clients to them when necessary. The complex therapeutic needs of
Hispanic clients challenge mental health professionals to update their
knowledge and skills continually. Occasionally, a clinician will need to
assist other mental health professionals who do not have a strong knowledge of minority cultures. This might involve acting as a facilitator between
the clients and other professionals in terms of clear communication and
the establishment of a professional relationship.

The following two therapeutic techniques are instrumental in the assessment phase. The World Test (World View Group, 1995) consists of a
series of circles of different sizes in which a client writes his or her name
and names of significant people in his or her life, positioned according to
closeness to the client. The Play Genogram (Gil & Sobol, 2003) asks the client to choose a miniature that represents his or her thoughts and feelings
about each family member, including him- or herself, and to place them in
a genogram that the therapist has drawn on a large piece of paper. A variation of this technique (developed by one of us, D. B.) is the Family Art
Genogram, which replaces the miniatures with symbolic drawings. It is
similar to the family portrait in the Family Art Evaluation (Kwiatkowska,
1978).

Hispanic children tend to present themes of community and closeness
with extended family members more frequently than white non-Hispanic
children do. For example, in the World Test and Family Play Genogram,
they include grandparents, uncles, aunts, cousins, nieces, and nephews, in
addition to the nuclear family members. Therapists from mainstream culture may erroneously interpret this phenomenon as family enmeshment
or lack of boundaries. It cannot be emphasized enough that closeness with
community and family is a core value of Hispanic culture. Consulting with

each other before making decisions, paying frequent visits, and showing respect for the elders are part of social codes in this culture (Falicov, 1998).

One of us (V. H.) has created techniques that address ethnic identity and expression of feelings. The first technique reinforces ethnic identity through identification with a positive role model. The therapist and the child watch a musical video of his or her favorite Hispanic singer. Next, the therapist invites the child to sing, dance, and act like the artist. During the interactions, the therapist highlights the Hispanic characteristics of the artist, as well as his or her spiritual and community values. It is important to expose minority children to role models from their culture, which are not readily available in the majority culture in which they are immersed. Currently, Hispanic musicians and other artists are enjoying great popularity, providing many more role models for Hispanic children.

The second technique, called Funny Faces, consists of the child's and therapist's showing each other feelings through facial expressions. This intervention offers several benefits: The child expresses a large range of feelings, due to relaxing while playing; it gives the child a sense of mastery from doing the task well; and it develops strong rapport with the therapist, as both are doing the same activity (making faces of feelings). It may be useful to take Polaroid pictures of these facial expressions, for future work on identification and expression of affect.

Other techniques, such as stress reduction through relaxation, are particularly necessary for traumatized children, as these techniques help them to reduce anxiety and fears. In our experience, Hispanic boys consider relaxation a "girls' matter" and are generally reluctant to learn and practice relaxation. However, they are more willing to learn breathing and visualization techniques. When we have used the technique involving visualization of a safe place, we have found it interesting that most boys choose as their safe environments everyday places, such as school and their bedrooms, whereas girls tend to choose outdoor settings, like the beach and the mountains.

As the termination of treatment approaches, we often ask clients to reflect on what they have learned in therapy, using any form of artistic expression. It is important to provide a free range of media in order to stimulate creativity. Some clients write messages on poster board; others make drawings or use miniatures symbolizing thoughts and feelings. When clients prefer to speak, we take notes and document what clients say. Next, each client builds a container to hold the artistic creations and to take them home—once again, to reinforce the transfer of knowledge from the therapeutic to the everyday context.

All materials used in the play therapy room must represent a variety of people and elements of different cultures. For work with Hispanic clients, it is necessary to have dolls with a variety of skin tones and features, so that all children can feel familiar and comfortable. The type of doll a child identifies with will depend on his or her acculturation level, as well as the child's own appearance. The physique of Hispanics is a complex mix of races; Central Americans can look very different from South Americans, and both can be dissimilar from Hispanic people of European or Caribbean origin. Even within countries, physical appearance varies based on ethnicity, geographical region, and background. Keeping such differences in mind is fundamental for respectful and useful therapeutic work.

In addition to human toys, one must have toys representing cultural elements, such as typical foods, transportation, infrastructure, mythical and popular characters, and others. It is difficult to provide cultural elements without falling into cultural stereotypes, such as the automatic association of tacos and burritos with Mexicans. Avoiding stereotypes is equally necessary for conveying respect to the clients. The same concepts apply to puppets, sandtray miniatures, and other toys.

Finally, no culturally sensitive play therapy room is complete without materials that stimulate creativity and freedom of expression in children and adults alike. Some examples are clay, textiles, scrap papers, paints, shells, rocks, feathers, and any colorful objects that may contribute to the precious process of creation.

CONCLUSION

Therapeutic work with culturally diverse populations requires mental health professionals to be educated about their clients' culture, as well as its interplay with the therapeutic context. Prominent issues and needs of Hispanic clients have been presented in this chapter—namely, significant family cohesion and closed family systems, *machismo*, hierarchical patterns, overcompliance (vs. agreement) with authority figures, extreme homophobia, reluctance to seek and/or receive therapy, unequal acculturation levels of family members, and intergroup racism.

As the case study has illustrated, many Hispanic families of sexually abused children tend to react to the disclosure of the abuse with anger in the case of fathers, and sorrow in the case of mothers. Certain degrees of family privacy, male dominance, and initial mistrust of the therapist are typical in the initial stages of treatment. Unfortunately, these cultural obstacles add to the obstacle created by the insufficient number of culturally competent mental health services. For treatment to be effective, it is necessary to empathize with the family's feelings, and to honor values such as family hierarchy and respect for authority.

Through our experiences with Hispanic families, we have realized that an integrative approach, including individual, group, and family therapy, seems to be the most successful with sexually abused Hispanic children. Involving the family in a child's treatment is particularly crucial, given the prominence of family interdependence in Hispanic culture. In addition, interventions need to take into account the client's extended family and community.

Therapists working with Hispanic families must incessantly be in tune with the culture of their clients, as well as provide a therapeutic environment that embraces both diversity and uniqueness. Honoring the clients' culture and supporting their cultural expression with appropriate therapeutic interventions and materials can accomplish this.

REFERENCES

Achenbach, T. M. (1991). *Child Behavior Checklist*. Burlington: University of Vermont, Department of Psychiatry.

Achenbach, T. M. (1991). *Child Behavior Checklist* [Spanish version]. Burlington: University of Vermont, Department of Psychiatry.

Briere, J. (1995). *Trauma Symptom Checklist for Children*. Odessa, FL: Psychological Assessment Resources.

Briere, J. (1995). *Trauma Symptom Checklist for Children* [Spanish version]. Odessa, FL: Psychological Assessment Resources.

Costantino, G., Malgady, R. G., & Rogler, L. H. (1986). *Cuento* therapy: A culturally sensitive modality for Puerto Rican children. *Journal of Consulting and Clinical Psychology, 54*(5), 639–645.

Falicov, C. J. (1998). *Latino families in therapy: A guide to multicultural practice*. New York: Guilford Press.

Fontes, L. A., Cruz, M., & Tabachnick, J. (2001). Views of sexual abuse in two cultural communities: An exploratory study among African Americans and Latinos. *Child Maltreatment, 6*(2), 103–117.

Friedrich, W. (1995). *Psychotherapy with sexually abused boys: An integrated approach*. Thousand Oaks, CA: Sage.

Gil, E. (1991). *The healing power of play*. New York: Guilford Press.

Gil, E. (1994). *Play in family therapy*. New York: Guilford Press.

Gil, E. (1996a). *Systemic treatment of families who abuse*. San Francisco: Jossey-Bass.

Gil, E. (1996b). *Treating abused adolescents*. New York: Guilford Press.

Gil, E., & Sobol, B. (2003). Engaging families in therapeutic play. In C. E. Bailey (Ed.), *Children in therapy: Using the family as a resource* (pp. 341–382). New York: Norton.

Grubbs, G. A. (1994). An abused child's use of sandplay in the healing process. *Clinical Social Work Journal, 22*(2), 193–209.

Ho, M. K. (1992). *Minority children and adolescents in therapy*. Newbury Park, CA: Sage.

Homeyer, L. E., & Landreth, G. L. (1998). Play behaviors of sexually abused children. *International Journal of Play Therapy, 4*(1), 49–71.

Johnston, S. S. M. (1997). The use of art and play therapy with victims of sexual abuse: A review of the literature. *Family Therapy, 24*(2), 101–113.

Kaduson, H., & Schaefer, C. (Eds.). (1997). *101 favorite play therapy techniques.* Northvale, NJ: Aronson.

Koss-Chioino, J., & Vargas, L. (1999). *Working with Latino youth: Culture, development and context.* San Francisco: Jossey-Bass.

Kwiatkowska, H. (1978). *Family therapy and evaluation through art.* Springfield, IL: Thomas.

Malchiodi, C. A. (1997). *Breaking the silence: Art therapy with children from violent homes* (2nd ed.). Bristol, PA: Brunner/Mazel.

Martinez, K. J., & Valdez, D. M. (1992). Cultural considerations in play therapy with Hispanic children. In L. A. Vargas & J. D. Koss-Chionio (Eds.), *Working with culture: Psychotherapeutic interventions with ethnic minority children and adolescents* (pp. 85–102). San Francisco: Jossey-Bass.

Mitchell, J. G. (Producer). (1995). *Super cachorro: Había una vez un sentimiento* [Videotape, Spanish version]. (Available from P.O. Box 2438, Sebastopol, CA 95473)

MTI/Film & Video (Producer). (1995). *Sooper puppy: Once upon a feeling* [Videotape]. (Available from 420 Academy Drive, Northbrook, IL 60062)

Pifalo, T. (2002). Pulling out the thorns: Art therapy with sexually abused children and adolescents. *Art Therapy: Journal of the American Art Therapy Association, 19*(1), 12–22.

Sexual abuse treatment: Status of the research. (2002, Winter). *Virginia Child Protection Newsletter, 63,* 14–15.

Shapiro, A. (Producer). (1994). *Break the silence: Kids against child abuse* [Videotape]. (Available from Aims Multimedia, 7910 DeSoto Avenue, Chatswoth, CA 91311-4409)

Sluzski, C. (1979). Migration and family conflict. *Family Process, 18*(4), 379–390.

Sue, D. W., & Sue, D. (1999). *Counseling the culturally different: Theory and practice* (3rd ed.). New York: Wiley.

Trostle, S. L. (1988). The effects of child-centered group play sessions on the social-emotional growth of three-to-six year old Puerto Rican children. *Journal of Research in Childhood Education, 3*(2), 93–106.

World View Group. (1995). *World Test.* Portland, OR: Author.

Wright, L. B., & Loiselle, M. (1997). *Back on track.* Brandon, VT: Safer Society Press.

7

❧

Musings on Working
with Native American Children
in Play Therapy

GERI GLOVER

My professional experience with Native peoples is varied, but limited. I have practiced filial therapy with families on the Flathead Reservation in northern Montana. I have seen children from the Pueblos of New Mexico, and "urban" Natives from several different tribes. I currently work with children and youth on the Alamo Navajo Reservation—a small community in central New Mexico, isolated from the big Navajo Reservation of western New Mexico and eastern Arizona.

Working with Native American clients and their families is as varied as working with any other population is. Of course, there are consistencies within tribes, and it is advisable that any therapist become well acquainted with the particular tribe or tribes seen most often. There are over 500 registered tribes in the United States. This is only the beginning of the variety found within and between tribes. Within every tribe, there are varying levels of acculturation. There are varying levels of Native language usage. There is intermarriage both between tribes and with other ethnicities. Although all Native Americans share a common history of oppression and discrimination, tribal beliefs and customs vary, as does individual adherence to those beliefs. Some Native Americans have become completely assimilated into the mainstream culture. Others maintain their traditional ways, which have been fairly consistent for centuries. For still others, poverty, alcoholism, and diseases have created dysfunctional family systems that appear to have no cultural foundation at all.

HISTORICAL EVENTS AND THEIR EFFECTS ON NATIVE AMERICANS

Almost from the beginning of European settlement in North America, but especially in the 19th and 20th centuries, various efforts were made to eliminate or change the many tribal cultures. No therapist should underestimate the current impact of historical trauma, and in order to understand Native Americans, it is first necessary to look at that history. According to the 2000 census figures, approximately 4.1 million people now consider themselves to be members of, or affiliated with, one of the more than 500 different Native American tribes (U.S. Bureau of the Census, 2002). Of this figure, 2.5 million report only Native American ancestry. The Native American population is growing, but Native Americans continue to represent less than 1% of the total U.S. population and are the smallest of the five major culture groups.

The Removal Policy of 1835 forced Native Americans to "Indian territory"—land that was often unproductive with few natural resources. The few resources that were available for farming or grazing quickly became overworked. Without an understanding of conservation, crop rotation, and irrigation, many reservations became wastelands. My father's relatives were moved from their beloved Bitterroot Valley to the Mission Valley. The Mission Valley was just as beautiful, but the land was rocky and difficult to farm.

The Dawes Severalty Act of 1837 then allotted each member of a Native American tribe, according to age, a specific portion of land. This allotment system took approximately 140 million acres of land treated to the Natives and reduced it to 50 million acres, with the excess land made available to settlers (Monahan, 1981). The hope was that Native Americans would accept individual land holdings and would be completely assimilated. My grandparents were affected by this act, and the consequences were disastrous. Even by the early 1900s, Native Americans had not developed a strong understanding of land ownership. This made them targets for unscrupulous people. The bank came in and gave credit to my grandparents, using their land as collateral. My grandparents, having no consistent source of income, were unable to pay the mortgage and lost their land to the bank, who in turn sold it to settlers from the dominant culture.

Off-reservation boarding schools were established in the United States in the late 1800s and exhibited their greatest growth in the 1920s. The schools were highly authoritative and were run in strict military fashion

(National Indian Child Abuse and Neglect Resource Center, 1980). The goal of education was to civilize and assimilate Native Americans into European American society (Reyhner, 1994). This plan for assimilation was not successful. Instead, those individuals who spent much of their childhood in boarding schools were deprived of an opportunity to experience family life. They reached adulthood without a clear concept of appropriate parenting behavior and family functioning. The boarding schools effectively destroyed the intergenerational transmission of family and parenting knowledge (George, 1997; Horejsi, Craig, & Pablo, 1992). These schools also introduced new and dysfunctional behaviors, such as the use of severe corporal punishment and sexual abuse.

In the 1950s, after World War II and the Korean conflict, the GI Bill and the Bureau of Indian Affairs Relocation Program for Job Training moved significant numbers of Native Americans to large urban areas. My father was sent to Chicago to learn a trade. He eventually returned to Montana and settled close to, but not on, his home reservation, as there were no jobs available there at that time.

The most recent interference in Native American life occurred from 1958 to 1968. The Child Welfare League of America supported the Indian Adoption Project (George, 1997). The league's philosophy was that the "forgotten child" on the reservation should be adopted and placed where there was less prejudice against Indians. In determining placement, the "best interests of the child" were to be considered. Poverty was judged a factor leading to neglect and abuse, and most Native Americans were poor. Middle-income Euopean American families were often chosen as the more beneficial placements. In 1978, this unprecedented removal of children from their families was halted by the Indian Child Welfare Act. I lost two cousins, whom I have never met, to this practice.

One of the results of these systematic efforts to eliminate or change Native American cultures has been the loss of Native languages. It is said that you can destroy a culture by taking away its language. Members of the tribes that live on the Flathead Reservation, and many others across the country, are working hard to recapture their languages. The Navajos have never lost theirs, and it is the first language for most of those living on the various Navajo Reservations. Although having Navajo as a first language may be positive in retaining culture, it has had a negative impact on the Navajos' ability to meet academic standards that are measured by tests written in English. The oral tradition, although adequate for centuries, is no longer the preferred method of disseminating information and knowledge. However, an emphasis on the importance of reading and writing has not risen to fill this void. The push to encourage parents to read to their young children is in its fledgling stage on the reservations.

This may appear at first to be a problem for the education system; however, in the United States, inadequate reading and writing skills in the English language contribute to the cycle of poverty and limited opportunities for Native Americans. Most reservations have few jobs, and many of those are limited to professionals with college degrees, such as teachers, nurses, doctors, counselors, accountants, and administrators. These professionals usually come in from outside the reservations, and being forced to depend on outsiders for services has an adverse effect on the self-esteem and motivation of the community members. At the same time, it relieves them from taking responsibility for the problems on their reservations, as they do not control their own programs.

Poverty, unemployment, and the high school dropout rate for Native Americans are all much higher than for the general population. Diabetes, alcoholism, heart disease, liver disease, suicide, and accidents all contribute to a short life expectancy of 44 years (Horejsi et al., 1992). More than one-third of all deaths occur among individuals under age 45, which is three times the rate for the general population of this age (Campbell, 1989).

These deaths result in an endless stream of funerals and grief (Horejsi, 1987). The emotional impact is even more intense because of the bonds by blood, marriage, and long friendships that typify Native American life. These frequent losses diminish people's coping capacity, as there is often no time to recover from a loss before another occurs. This may partially account for the high rate of depression among Native Americans (Indian Health Services, 1990). Another outcome of all these deaths is that many children have lost one or both of their parents. The extended family or "village" concept of child rearing is a natural way to have several adults involved in raising a child. However, this works best when there is at least one adult who claims the child. Problems develop when the child does not have that one champion, and being raised by the "village" becomes "It's your turn to deal with him or her."

TRADITIONAL NATIVE AMERICAN VALUES

Understanding traditional Native American values is important in order to provide the best services for Native Americans. Native American families are characterized as collective, cooperative social networks that reach from the mother and father to the extended family, to the community, to the tribe (Harrison, Wilson, Pine, Chan, & Buriel, 1990). Within this system, traditional values include generosity; respect for elders, for other people, and for all creation; harmony; and individual freedom.

In the dominant culture, where success is defined by wealth and possessions, it may be difficult to accept the values of simplicity, generosity, and nonmaterialism, but these values have helped to sustain the Native American people through generations of economic and personal hardship. Still, there has been a significant shift toward materialism in the last couple of generations. Native Americans are not immune to the constant barrage of advertising to buy this or that. Coupled with the long-held belief in living life on a day-to-day basis, there is sometimes little thought for the future. If you have money in your pocket, it should be spent. If your family or friends ask you for money, and you have some in your pocket, you give it to them. If your children ask for things and you have money in your pocket, you buy them things. The concept of saving the little money you have, so that it will grow into more money with which you could buy a car or house, is too far into the future and almost impossible to imagine. This way of life is not exclusive to Native Americans, but can be more widely understood as a result of generations of living in poverty.

Great respect is shown to the elders of a tribe. Young children are taught that age is a gift, a badge of honor (Burgess, 1980). To have grown old indicates that a person has done the right things, pleased the creator, and lived in tune with nature and others. In a traditional home, elders are expected to give advice and counsel. Grandparents teach about nature and tell stories of creation and culture. They have wisdom regarding order and balance, which they have learned from the mountains, rivers, trees, and wind. These structured teaching and learning experiences are supported by the parents and not interrupted. In a home that lacks the structure of either the traditional or the dominant culture, elders are not so highly revered. They are sought out primarily when things come undone, and in many ways their usefulness has become limited to serving as sources for child care and financial support.

Respect for others is a prominent traditional Native American value. The National Indian Child Abuse and Neglect Resource Center (1981) issued the following statement:

> Native American people have traditionally held a great respect for all peoples. We have a tradition of respect in our culture and in our spirituality. We respect the earth, elders, children, animals, all of life. We have lost some of this respect along with our languages and many of our customs. But it is not too late to maintain those which are left and to use traditional concepts of respect in raising children. (p. 6)

Harmony is valued, because of the belief that everything is related and it is important for all things to be in balance. Traditional Native Americans operate in a relational model that is intuitive, nontemporal, and fluid (Cross, 1998). Balance and harmony among multiple variables, including individual, family, community, nature, and metaphysical forces, are seen as necessary for health (Cross, 1998; Sanchez, Plawecki, & Plawecki, 1996). The weakness of this relational model is that it seeks harmony even at the expense of the individual (Cross, 1998).

The most controversial value is that of individual freedom or noninterference. Any person, even a young child, is free to make choices, but the person must accept responsibility for the choices made. In a traditional context, the correct choices have benefits for the family, friends, or the group. Autonomy is highly valued, and children are allowed to make their own decisions and operate semi-independently at an early age, with the freedom to experience natural consequences (LaFromboise & Graff Low, 1998). Just as for many who have been raised in the dominant culture, the natural consequences for poor choices are now more frightening than they were even a generation ago. The world is simply a more dangerous place, and this style of parenting may be more hazardous to the well-being of children. In the traditional family, a youth of about the age of 14 was welcomed into the community as an adult. In an isolated place where plenty of manual work was necessary simply to survive, this tradition was profitable for the tribe. In today's society, where adolescents are not required or expected to contribute to the family's survival, having the freedom and responsibility of adulthood at age 14 actually creates problems and causes strife in the family.

ISSUES IN TREATMENT OF NATIVE AMERICANS

In treatment, the level of acculturation once again becomes an issue. There must be harmony between the treatment and the person's degree of acculturation (Williams & Ellison, 1999). A more assimilated, nontraditional person is likely to choose the dominant culture's lifestyle and medicine. Indicators of this preference may be a relatively high level of formal education; minimal, if any, interaction with the reservation; less dependence on the extended family; and previous experience with Western medicine, either personally or within the immediate family.

In the traditional family, illness equals imbalance and is a function of the person's perception of being unable to fulfill traditional role obligations. An intervention is designed to restore physical well-being and harmony to damaged social and spiritual relationships. This is done by using ceremony and ritual; by consulting traditional healers; and by including peers, family, and community representatives in the intervention. Traditional Native Americans encountering the dominant culture's health care system feel frustrated that their powerful knowledge about how to care for an illness to mind, body, or spirit is not utilized as a legitimate avenue for healing.

In times past, a healer may have told an individual to make certain changes in his or her life in order to regain health. This was done in one or two visits, and the individual was expected to make those changes and all would be well. For Native Americans who remember traditional healers, but do not practice a traditional lifestyle, the responsibility of the person being healed has been forgotten. They go to a counselor believing that things will be fixed. The concept of going to counseling once a week for 30 minutes or an hour, over an extended period of time, is difficult to grasp. Making a drop-in visit without an appointment is still the preferred style of Native American clients. The present-time orientation is dominant, and they want relief from a problem when the problem occurs. This often feels like "crisis mode" for the therapist, and it makes it very difficult to be proactive and try to prevent negative consequences before they happen. In regard to children, though, this style is not unlike that of many parents from the dominant culture who bring their children to a therapist to be "straightened out" or "fixed" immediately.

To prepare for working with Native Americans, Weaver (1999) suggests that the practitioner learn as much as possible about important issues within the Native American population, but also be alert to individual differences. In addition to proactively taking the client's perspective, specific skills can be helpful in working with Native Americans. These include patience, the ability to tolerate and respect silences, listening, using humor, and being willing to be the target of humor (Weaver, 1999; Williams & Ellison, 1999). The practitioner must practice humility and show a desire to learn about the person's culture. Respect and a nonjudgmental ability to grasp a different worldview are also valuable skills.

As noted above, the history of Native Americans has left many families so highly disrupted and even disabled that many positive traditional ways have been forgotten (Burgess, 1980; National Indian Child Abuse and Neglect Resource Center, 1980). Still, some basic values remain common among Native American people, such as the importance of extended family relationships and support systems, nonmaterialism, health defined as being "balanced," and the concept of individual freedom within the framework of a harmonious and generous life. Specific traditions and practices (such as rites of passage and death/mourning rituals) differ greatly between tribes, and practitioners must learn these specifics with humility and an open mind. Traditional values are practiced by many Native peoples, but just as in the dominant culture, television, movies, music, computers, and electronic games have replaced many of the day-to-day activities of Native families. It takes a lot of work on the part of Native Americans to maintain a traditional life.

In therapy with children, actual play behaviors are not dissimilar to those of children from the dominant culture. Both girls and boys enjoy using art materials, easel painting, role playing (e.g., playing store), and creating scenes in the sand. Many girls are attracted to doll play and caring for babies. Many boys are attracted to aggressive play with action figures. Some children talk while they play, and others do not. In group play, children may speak in their tribal language rather than English. Verbal processing of difficult concepts may be slower for those children who do not speak English as a first language, but processing does occur in the play. As in therapy with children from all minority cultures, the therapist must be on guard not to assume that simply because a Native American child plays happily with the toys provided, the playroom is culturally appropriate. Cradleboards, dark-haired and dark-skinned dolls, musical instruments, traditional foods and utensils, and forest animals will give Native American children permission to bring culture into their play.

CASE EXAMPLE

A 3-year-old male Navajo boy was referred at age 3 because of aggressive behaviors in preschool. The boy's mother had been killed in an automobile accident when he was 2 years old. The child was in the vehicle at the time of the accident and was present at his mother's death. Because the father was unavailable to raise his son, a maternal great-aunt was given legal custody. Although the great-aunt is in her early 50s, she has little energy to deal with a headstrong preschooler who was traumatized at an early age.

The child was referred for aggressive behaviors in the preschool, including biting, hitting, yelling angrily at peers to "get away," shoving, and grabbing. He was not able to share toys with others, even with adult assistance. He was easily angered by other children who came into his space. If he fell or bumped something, he would immediately break into tears.

Therapeutic modalities selected for this child included consultation with the child's great-aunt and teachers, individual child-centered play therapy, and group play therapy in the classroom setting. In addition, interaction, under supervision if necessary, was encouraged between the father and his son. The mother's relatives were not willing to try this idea. They hoped that the father would simply disappear, as they thought he would have a negative influence on the child. Eventually there would be interaction between the father and his son, as this is unavoidable in a small Native community. It is unfortunate that the relationship could not be nurtured when the child was young.

The behavior plan arranged with the classroom teachers and special education teacher included activities for the child to learn give-and-take skills with an adult before introducing another child, and then only introducing one child at a time. In addition, the teachers were asked to continually remind the child to use words rather than hit other children. The teachers were encouraged to be vigilant, to "catch" the child before he made a mistake, and to help him work through the emotions that caused an angry outburst. In addition, teachers were encouaged to help the child learn when to take a break from the group. Not all children are suited to group day care situations; they become overstimulated and easily upset by the constant presence of many other young children and adults.

Individual child-centered play therapy is an appropriate choice for working with Native American children. Showing respect for the child and allowing the child self-direction are key factors in child-centered play therapy and these concepts support values held by traditional Native American parents. Unlike more behaviorally oriented therapies, this model of play therapy is not directed toward specific problems, but is generic in nature. It is conducted in a present-oriented fashion, allowing the child to communicate thoughts, needs, and feelings at the moment they occur. Both verbal and nonverbal communication are acceptable and valued. Feelings such as frustration, anger, fear of abandonment, or concerns about personal safety, which manifest in inappropriate and maladaptive behaviors, can be addressed through encouraging the child to play them out in the safe, interpersonal atmosphere of a play session and in the presence of a warm, caring adult. Play is the primary way in which children express themselves, grow, and develop. Play also improves socialization and interpersonal skills.

Minimal time was required to develop a relationship with this particular child as he seemed to crave individual adult attention, the cornerstone of child-centered play therapy. Once contact was established, the playroom setting provided substantial opportunities for the child to express himself. The environment included typical preschool materials such as paints, paper, blocks, farm and zoo animals, a dollhouse, cars, and a housekeeping center. In addition, dark-skinned and dark-haired dolls, a traditional Navajo cradleboard, blankets, Native American dollhouse figures, and a drum were available for play. The farm animals included several horses, sheep, and goats. The playroom walls displayed many representations of Navajo culture and people.

During the first few sessions, the child spent time exploring the playroom and becoming acquainted with the variety of toys available. He eventually settled into a routine of caring for the babies and playing in the housekeeping center. This is typical play for preschoolers as it is often their most significant experience. Families spend a great deal of time preparing meals and caring for children. Although caring for babies is a nurturing activity, this child often shifted between gentleness and aggressiveness. There was obvious ambivalence about how small people can and should be treated. These activities gave the therapist many opportunities to respond to feelings of caring, anger, frustration, and confusion. With consistent responses and unconditional acceptance of these various feelings, the child began to learn that his feelings were valid and that he was valued. Although his feelings were always accepted, at times, when the play became too destructive, the therapist would set a limit: For example, "I know you are angry that the baby keeps crying, but the baby is not for throwing at the window. You can throw it on the pillow." Limits on behavior were only necessary when the child accelerated to a point of hurting himself, breaking the toys, or hurting the therapist.

Techniques in child-centered play therapy include being fully present with the child, responding to the child's behaviors and feelings, and setting limits on behavior only when necessary. The child chooses to play or not to play. The child chooses to speak or not to speak. The child leads and the therapist follows. When children become disruptive in a preschool setting, adults often become more strict. Rather than helping the child to learn how to control their own behavior, they attempt to control the child. Individual play therapy sessions allowed this child to experience self-control. He began to develop the ability to control the escalation of rising emotions as he experienced them rather than having them cut short by an adult who found his emotions unacceptable. He learned that certain behaviors were not allowed, but that any emotion was valid.

Group play therapy in the classroom setting provided additional experiences in a controlled environment for the child to practice appropriate behaviors. He participated in group play therapy with one other child of the same age. During these sessions, the child was required to share the attention of the therapist. Conflicts inevitably arose and the therapist was able to model appropriate behavior during these conflicts. Techniques for child-centered group play therapy are identical to those for individual child-centered play therapy. The therapist is present with the children, responds to their actions and feelings, and sets limits when necessary. The play is directed by the children.

Both individual child-centered play therapy and group play therapy occurred weekly for a period of 4 months. During this time, the child developed more self-control and became less sensitve to the typical bumps and falls of early childhood. Biting was almost eliminated, and yelling at peers was reduced considerably. The child continued to have angry outbursts, but the level of aggressiveness was reduced. The child particpated in group play for short periods of time, but continued to become more easily tired and moody than is typical for children of this age. Learning this child's particular temperament was essential to make this child's time in preschool less stressful for everyone. It is important also to be aware that this child, who experienced great trauma and loss at an early age, will need continued support as he negotiates the various milestones of his life and as he views the traumatic experience from perspectives changed by age.

SUMMARY

Working with children and families from Native American cultures is challenging. Many of the difficulties Native Americans suffered in the past continue to influence their descendants today. Generations of poverty, language challenges, and lack of control over their own lives have contributed to the current conditions within many tribes. Only recently have Native Americans, as a group, challenged the status quo and made strides in changing a situation over which they previously had no control. Let us hope that in the years to come, the dysfunctional Native American family will be the exception rather than the rule, and the positive values shared by Native Americans will be a model for the dominant culture.

REFERENCES

Burgess, B. J. (1980). Parenting in the Native-American community. In M. D. Fantini & R. Cárdenas (Eds.), *Parenting in a multicultural society* (pp. 63–73). New York: Longman.

Campbell, G. (1989). The political epidemiology of infant mortality. *American Indian Culture and Research Journal, 13*(3), 1–20.

Cross, T. L. (1998). The world view of American Indian families. In Child Welfare League of America (Ed.), *Culturally competent practice: A series from Children's Voice magazine* (pp. 23–31). Washington, DC: Child Welfare League of America Press.

George, L. J. (1997). Why the need for the Indian Child Welfare Act? In G. R. Anderson, A. Shea Ryan, & B. R. Leashore (Eds.), *The challenge of permanency planning in a multicultural society* (pp. 165–175). Binghamton, NY: Haworth Press.

Harrison, A. O., Wilson, M. N., Pine, C. J., Chan, S. Q., & Buriel, R. (1990). Family ecologies of ethnic minority children. *Child Development, 61*, 347–362.

Horejsi, C. (1987). *Child welfare practice and the Native American family in Montana: A handbook for social workers*. Missoula: University of Montana.

Horejsi, C., Craig, B. H. R., & Pablo, J. (1992). Reactions by Native American parents to child protection agencies: Cultural and community factors. *Child Welfare, 66*(4), 329–342.

Indian Health Services. (1990). *National Plan for Native American Mental Health Services*. Rockville, MD: Author.

LaFromboise, T. D., & Graff Low, K. (1998). American Indian children and adolescents. In J. T. Gibbs, L. N. Huang, & Associates, *Children of color: Psychological interventions with culturally diverse youth* (pp. 112–142). San Francisco: Jossey-Bass.

Monahan, T. C. (1981). *An exploratory study of selected characteristics of parent committees associated with projects funded under Title IV, Public Law 92-318, The Indian Education Act, Part A*. New Brunswick, NJ: Rutgers University.

National Indian Child Abuse and Neglect Resource Center. (1980). *Indian culture and its relationship to child abuse and neglect. Revised.* Tulsa, OK: Author. (ERIC Document Reproduction Service No. ED 229 193)

National Indian Child Abuse and Neglect Resource Center. (1981). *Parenting education: Discipline skills.* Tulsa, OK: Author. (ERIC Document Reproduction Service No. ED 229 199)

Reyhner, J. (1994). *American Indian/Alaska Native education.* Bloomington, IN: Phi Delta Kappa Educational Foundation. (ERIC Document Reproduction Service No. ED 369 585)

Sanchez, T. R., Plawecki, J. A., & Plawecki, H. M. (1996). The delivery of culturally sensitive health care to Native Americans. *Journal of Holistic Nursing, 14*(4), 295–307.

U.S. Bureau of the Census. (2002, February). *The American Indian and Alaska Native population: 2000.* Washington, DC: U.S. Department of Commerce.

Weaver, H. N. (1999). Indigenous people and the social work profession: Defining culturally competent services. *Social Work, 44*(3), 217–225.

Williams, E. E., & Ellison, F. (1999). Culturally informed social work practice with American Indian clients: Guidelines for non-Indian social workers. In P. L. Ewalt, E. M. Freeman, A. E. Fortune, D. L. Poole, & S. L. Witkin (Eds.), *Multicultural issues in social work: Practice and research* (pp. 78–84). Washington, DC: National Association of Social Workers.

8

❧

Play Therapy
with Asian Children

SHU-CHEN KAO

The importance of cultural considerations has already been acknowledged in the field of play therapy. Gaining cultural sensitivity is an ongoing process for all play therapists; it begins with self-exploration and awareness, and continues with the acquisition of knowledge and skills. The greater the extent to which a therapist knows the symbols, meanings, and messages of a child's culture, the greater the therapist's ability to achieve cross-cultural identification will be (Glover, 2001). In order to explore the complexities of communication with Asian children and their families, this chapter describes some common characteristics and values of Asian cultures—with a focus on Chinese culture—that affect their communication behaviors. The terms "Asian" and "Chinese" are both used in this chapter. The use of "Asian" implies that a concept is applicable to various Asian cultures; when the word "Chinese" is used, the concept is limited to the Chinese population. Some specific suggestions and reminders for play therapists are offered to facilitate better communication with Asian children and parents.

THE ASIAN AMERICAN
POPULATION: BACKGROUND

Since the 1960s, the Asian American population has been one of the fastest-growing ethnic groups in the United States (Vardell, 1996). The 1990 U.S.

Census report indicated that there were 7.3 million Asian Americans in the country at that time. The trend of increasing Asian immigration has drastically increased the enrollment of Asian students in U.S. schools (Huang, 1993). Asians are a very large and diverse group, composed of at least 53 different ethnic groups (Pagani-Tousignant, 1992). Lee and Childress (1999) have identified four large general ethnic groupings within the Asian community:

1. *Pacific Islanders*—primarily people from Hawaii, Samoa, and Guam.
2. *Southeast Asians*—primarily people from Vietnam, Thailand, Cambodia, Laos, and Myanmar (formerly Burma), but also people from the Philippines, Singapore, Malaysia, and Indonesia.
3. *East Asians*—people from China, Japan, and Korea.
4. *South Asians*—people from India, Pakistan, and Sri Lanka.

Not only do these four large groups differ in sociocultural traits, but subgroups within each group often differ as well. It is important not to generalize an understanding of one group to another (Huang, 1993). The four large groups represent a wide range of educational, linguistic, economic, occupational, and cultural backgrounds. Each of them, and the individual subgroups within each one, deserve specific recognition.

The common cultural threads running through Asian cultures are often so strong that they are maintained for generations after people move to another country. Play therapists must identify such differences to devise appropriate communication strategies for counseling Asian children (Kong, 1985). However, because each group has its own distinctive cultural background, unique historical experiences, and reasons for immigration, it is difficult if not impossible to make sweeping generalizations about Asian Americans. In this chapter, as noted earlier, Chinese culture is the focus of discussion. The exploration of the topic of play therapy with Chinese children aims at facilitating play therapists' awareness and generating ideas for appropriate adaptation in play therapy. Furthermore, it may serve as an example for modifying play therapy to other Asian cultures.

Characteristics that distinguish Chinese American culture from the dominant European American culture are collectivism, future goal orientation, the importance of the extended family, shame and face-saving reactions, pressure for academic achievement, authoritarian and patriarchal family structures, permissive child rearing in early childhood, and authoritarian child rearing in middle to later childhood (Manery, 2000). A basic knowledge of a child's heritage should be in the background of the therapist's awareness, while the child's particular needs and idiosyncrasies should be in the foreground.

CHINESE CULTURAL
AND COMMUNICATION ISSUES
AFFECTING THE PLAY THERAPY PROCESS

Values and norms embedded in language, religion, philosophy, custom, and social organizations, such as the strong emphasis on the family, are important variables affecting Asian Americans' behaviors. For example, under the influence of Chinese Confucianism, East Asians developed complex literate cultures and cohesive family organizations. Socioeconomic status and immigration history, often related to cultural differences, also affect Asian Americans' communication and life adjustment (Hall, 1977). In working with Asian children, a play therapist will see the child in the play session and parents in the consultation session. The following are some cultural and communication issues that may arise in the play therapy process with Asian families in general and Chinese families in particular.

Views of Children and Childhood

Traditionally, Asian children are viewed as "little adults." They are expected to be well-behaved and hard-working. The family unit is so strong that children are not encouraged to be independent from parents and family. Because children are the hope for the family, parents impose pressure on their children. The family structure is not only authoritarian, but patriarchal: Boys are usually valued over girls, because boys carry the family name and are expected to bring honor to the family. Childhood is viewed as a preparation period for adulthood; therefore, working hard for academic performance (see "Academic Expectations," below) and learning survival skills for real life are important.

Views of Toys and Play

Most traditional and popular toys in Asian culture can be divided into five major categories: physical, social, intellectual, seasonal, and gambling play. Chinese parents prefer toys that have educational purposes, and they approve of children's play when they see the educational value of the specific play activity. An old Chinese saying—"Advancement in achievement comes from hard work, and deterioration in achievement comes from play"—reflects the traditional discouragement of children's play in this culture. The efforts of early childhood educators in recent decades have been aimed at changing parents' view of play by claiming that very young children learn best through play. Today, most parents are able to appreciate the value of play in early childhood. For school-age children, however, parents are not completely convinced about the value of play; parents still tend to focus on goal-oriented activities for children of this age.

Gender differences also exist in the traditional selection of toys and play activities for Chinese children. Boys are encouraged to engage in physical, aggressive, and constructional toys and activities, while girls are encouraged to engage in calm, nurturing, pretend/fantasy toys and activities. Boys are allowed to use more space in play and to participate in more outdoor play (Kuo, 1992). Although these gender differences continue to exist in the culture, the emphasis on gender equality is narrowing the gap gradually. With the progress in international trade, mass communication, and electronic commerce, children in Western and Eastern cultures also share similar exposure to new trends in toys, especially in computer games.

The Parent–Child Relationship

As noted above, the fundamental unit in Asian cultures is the family, as opposed to the individual in the West. The most important interpersonal relationships in the society are within the family. There is an emphasis on the unquestionable authority of parents and the expectation of obedience from children. Parents' authoritarian role is played out by keeping the family protected and children controlled. These cultures emphasize a close bond within the family and do not appreciate early independence and separation. Pressures may also come from adults who are members of the extended family or close friends to control children's behaviors. In Western culture, the interrelatedness of the nuclear and extended family may be misunderstood as codependence or other family pathology.

Shame and Face-Saving Reactions

Shame has a predominant influence in traditional Asian cultures. In these cultures, people learn to act very cautiously, because an individual's misbehavior reflects badly upon the status of the family and community (Sue & Sue, 2002). In a play session, a child may be cautious and may not play or talk spontaneously. This behavior may be misunderstood as resistance to the therapy. It is important for the therapist to entertain the possibility that the child may be acting under the influence of having to present him- or herself as "a good kid from a prestigious family." Similar misunderstanding may exist in interpreting a parent's response in the consultation session. Common nonverbal behaviors seen in Chinese parents (e.g., smiling, head nodding, and verbal assent) may represent friendliness and interest, while holding back from direct sharing. These nonverbal behaviors may be interpreted as agreement by a Western therapist. It is important to observe both parents and children carefully and remain open-minded about the possible meaning of such behaviors. Appropriate clarification may be used to enhance accurate interpretation of the communication. In addition, encouraging and directive statements may guide the parents to open up. The following are examples:

- "I can help your child better if I know what's really on your mind."
- "Please trust me that I would just like to understand more, and that I am not going to judge anyone here."
- "We are in the same boat: We want to help your child. Don't feel embarrassed to let me know your thoughts and worries."

Views of Mental Illness and Psychotherapy

There is an entrenched belief shared by Asians that psychological distress is a manifestation of organic disorders (Kleinman & Good, 1985). Asian Americans often view mental illness as a personal weakness that can be controlled by disciplining one's thinking and avoiding morbid thoughts, rather than sharing this weakness with a stranger. This view is compounded by the concern about bringing shame to the family, mentioned above. As a result, professional help may be sought only as a last resort, when the problems are extremely serious, or when family and community resources have been exhausted (Morrissey, 1997). The myth that Asian Americans are a "model minority" has caused additional problems for members of the Asian community, as they set unrealistic expectations for themselves, and this label may have hindered them in seeking and accepting psychotherapy and other social services (Vardell, 1996). A sensitive understanding of their anxiety, and warm support for their uncertainty, will be necessary in building a relationship with Asian parents and children. *A Child's First Book about Play Therapy* (Nemiroff & Annunziata, 1990) is a great way of introducing play therapy to parents and children. Furthermore, offering information about child psychopathology can enhance parents' knowledge of their child's problem.

Language Barriers

Language barriers may force both parents and children to choose simple words that fail to express complex thoughts and feelings (Sue & Sue, 2002). Play therapists who have no knowledge of a family's mother tongue may use simple and easy language to encourage clients' understanding and communication. The nature of play therapy in a particular case may help to reduce the language barriers for a child. For parent consultation, depending on the parents' educational status and immigration history, help from an interpreter may be needed. If so, it is important to find an appropriate interpreter. In daily life, older children and teenagers who have acquired competence in English often serve as interpreters for their families. In parent consultation, however, there may be a role conflict for a child or teenager who has the traditional obedient role of an offspring and the more powerful role as an interpreter. In addition, some therapy issues will not be appropriate to discuss in front of a child.

Academic Expectations

Similar to middle- and upper-income European Americans, East Asians, particularly the Chinese, highly value formal education. Children's performance in school is directly related to the family's prestige: High achievement brings honor and prestige to the family, whereas failure brings shame (Lee, 1989; Shen & Mo, 1990). With such a belief, it is understandable that parents exert a lot of pressure on children to work hard and to achieve in school. Such pressure may lead to problems for children, including constant self-criticism and lowered self-esteem even if they attain relatively high levels of success, and shame and alienation if they fail to achieve as expected (Csikszentmihalyi, 1997). Parents of children who struggle may also suffer, as they interpret their children's school failure as their own parenting failure and feel desperate for the family's future. The academic issues need to be discussed openly in the therapy process, so that the underlying family issues can be understood.

Relationship with Authority Figures

Asian parents tend to have high expectation and respect for teachers, as they have authority over their children's schooling. And such parents are likely to view not only teachers, but therapists, as professionals with authority. Being sensitive to these expectations will help make it easier for Asian parents to talk in therapy about their children's school problems. Therapists' patience and explanation about the tenets of play therapy will be helpful. Because of their respect for authority figures, Asian parents tend to be cautious at the beginning of a relationship. In the initial session, discussion may proceed as if everyone is in accord, until finally the parents are asked (and may refuse) to demonstrate approval by signing an agreement (Matsuda, 1989). Being patient, with an open and inviting attitude, usually helps Asian parents to become more comfortable and open with authority figures.

Suggestions for the Parent Consultation Process

Based on the discussion above, some tentative suggestions for play therapists about consulting with Asian parents in general and Chinese parents in particular are as follows:

1. *Building a cooperative working relationship.* Bonding between Asian parents and children is strong. Therapists should thus respect the family bond and be cautious about judging it from a Western cultural perspective. However, many Asian parents are eager to know more about how play therapy may help their children, and successful cooperation with parents can be facilitated by devoting time and effort to parent consultation. Indeed, involving parents is crucial for a successful intervention, because the family offers strong support as part of the network of change. Parents also need help in understanding and trusting the play therapy process. A play therapist needs to be patient with parents, attentive to nonverbal cues, and comfortable with periods of silence (which may be used by parents to reflect on what has been said).

2. *Providing support for parents.* A therapist can demonstrate support for parents by being willing to listen to the parents' complaints about cultural adjustment, especially if they are new immigrants. Showing interest in the parents' culture through asking and talking about the culture will also help to build a positive relationship. It is important to respect cultural beliefs and, as much as possible, to incorporate them into therapy. Many Asian parents come into therapy without knowing what to expect (Morrissey, 1997); therefore, providing basic information about therapy is important. Expressing care and concern about the parents' feelings (threats to cultural identity, powerlessness, feelings of marginality, loneliness, hostility, alienation, discrimination, etc.) can ease them into the consultation process.

3. *Discussing the child.* Asian parents tend to expect the therapist to provide education; parent consultation may thus include some parenting education. Establishing the therapist's professional role and assuming appropriate authority to build up parents' trust and hope for the therapy may also be appropriate strategies, since traditional Asian parents may expect and prefer a direct, active, and authoritative approach on the part of the therapist. It will be helpful to provide clear and full information, such as what will be provided by the therapist and what is expected from the parents in the therapy. It will also be helpful to encourage parents to share opinions and concerns openly, and to express value for what they have said.

4. *Handling academic concerns.* Academic achievement is usually a crucial topic in a parent consultation because of the family's commitment to education. Combining academic concerns with a child's adjustment issues will be a good strategy in work with Chinese parents. In the counseling process, the child's wishes or decisions may conflict with the parents' or family's expectations. The play therapist may help the child and parents come to a comfortable compromise so that family harmony can be maintained.

PLAY THERAPY MATERIALS

Many play therapy materials recommended in the Western literature (Kottman, 2001; Landreth, 1991) are cross-cultural in nature. However, thoughtful consideration of particular materials for children from a specific cultural background may be helpful. For example, a colleague and I (Kao & Landreth, 2001) have suggested some modifications for Chinese children. Our recommendations include providing school supplies for playing out academic-related themes; substituting traditional toys for, or adding them to, similar-purpose Western toys; using culturally appropriate kitchen and table materials to reenact real-life home situations; and using Asian figures, puppets, and dolls to replace typical Western figures.

Play therapists who employ sandtray techniques in the play sessions may need to make an extra effort to understand how the miniatures used in such play vary in symbolic meanings for children from different ethnic backgrounds. For instance, I have seen European American children use a black sheep to represent their role in their families, but the black sheep does not have the same meaning in Asian cultures. In addition, as with toys, miniatures specific to various aspects of Asian culture will be helpful—for example, human figures, religious figures, buildings, and so forth. Finally, it is important to remember that the ultimate key to symbolic meanings of miniatures lies in the individual child's mind.

Indeed, being open-minded is important in understanding the symbolic meaning of any type of play. A play therapist may take common play themes for granted, while missing a double meaning that may arise from a different cultural context or from an individual child's situation. A careful observation and understanding of these factors will be very helpful.

SUGGESTIONS FOR MODIFYING PLAY THERAPY TECHNIQUES

I believe that although the fundamental principles in counseling—including being genuine, consistent, caring, and accepting—are universal across cultures, some play therapy techniques may be modified to better meet the needs and issues of Asian children. It should, of course, be remembered that children coming to see a play therapist may have behaviors contradicting their group stereotypes; the play therapist should work to transcend such stereotypes and treat each child as a unique individual. With this caveat and with the fundamental principles I have mentioned in mind, I now provide some suggestions to stimulate play therapists' creativity in trying new techniques to enhance the therapeutic work.

Adjusting the Frequency of Tracking Behavior

For a child entering a new therapy relationship, a play therapist tends to use the tracking technique to establish a relationship and show that the therapist cares about and attempts to understand the child. Consideration should be given to the emphasis on collectivism in Asian cultures, however. To an Asian child, being part of a group may be more comfortable than being singled out. Frequent tracking may be experienced as excessive attention and may cause self-doubt in the child. Adjusting the frequency of tracking responses at the beginning of therapy, according to the child's need, may help the child feel more comfortable.

Clarifying the Nature of Limit Setting

The importance of limit setting for a therapeutic relationship cannot be over-emphasized. However, it is important to consider that some Asian children may be sensitive to criticism, because they may feel that they have done something to bring shame to their families. Limit setting that is clear and directed to a behavior, not to a child, will be useful in dealing with this possible sensitivity to criticism. It is also important to make sure that the child does not feel that he or she has lost face due to the limit setting. Presenting a limit as a rule may prevent the child from taking it too personally.

Being Attentive and Sensitive to Nonverbal Cues

Asian children are frequently viewed as quiet, polite, hard-working, and cooperative. However, language and cultural differences may present barriers in communication and limit a child's expression. Furthermore, self-expression, or voicing personal opinions that define and heighten the sense of oneself, is not seen as a desirable behavior (Dwivedi, 1999). These attitudes may also limit the child's spontaneous expression in the play session. If so, the therapist may need to pay more attention to nonverbal cues, to understand the underlying meaning of the child's play.

Being Careful about Reflection of Feelings

Asians are more reserved than most Westerners about expressing various feelings openly. It is expected that older children will learn to contain and regulate their own feelings; acting upon feelings without regard to others is seen as a sign of emotional immaturity. This may contrast with the typical focus in the therapy process on exploring deep underlying feelings. Caution should be taken by the therapist in choosing words to reflect a specific feeling. Consideration should be given to avoiding strong feeling words that may make the child feel awkward. The therapist may also learn to appreciate the covert affectionate behaviors within interactions.

Being Cautious in Interpreting Play Behavior

Understanding the symbolic meaning of play is a powerful way to promote insight. As noted earlier, the interpretation of play behavior may vary, depending on the therapist's unique cultural perspective. It is advisable to keep an open mind, use observations to generate hypotheses, and wait to gather further information before making an interpretation or coming up with an explanation. In addition, a therapist should always leave room for the child's correction of the therapist's interpretation, and should not automatically view this as the child's resistance to the therapy.

Taking a More Directive Approach

Many nondirective play therapists work effectively with Asian children. However, many Asian children are more familiar with adults' being authority figures and adopting an educational role. A child may need to be prepared by the therapist and given some clear indications of what to expect from play therapy. Thus a directive approach may be helpful in guiding the child into the therapy process.

Using More Self-Esteem-Building Skills

Encouragement is a useful tool in building a relationship with a child, as it communicates understanding and trust. Because a therapist is viewed as similar to a teacher (an authority figure from a Chinese point of view), children feel a sense of accomplishment when being recognized by an authority figure.

Communicating Genuineness and Trust through Nonverbal Skills

Communication between people goes beyond words. A play therapist can always express genuine care and trust through his or her face, gesture, voice, and so on. Both therapist and child can accept that cultural limitations exist and can acknowledge the efforts made in communication. The therapist's effort can be sensed by the child, and I believe that the child can change and grow in response to the adult's genuine care.

OTHER CONCERNS
IN THE THERAPY PROCESS

Culturally Sensitive Assessment

Practitioners who work with Asian children confront such fundamental issues as the cultural validity of the diagnostic tools and systems that are available to them. Many assessment instruments have not been normed on sufficient numbers of Asian children; some subgroups of Asian children may not be represented in the norms at all; and the tests may be culturally biased. The play therapist needs to be careful in the selection of the instrument and the interpretation of test scores in working with Asian children. Young children being exposed to their mother tongue at home and English in day care/preschool may be delayed in their English-language development. It is therefore important to be cautious in making judgments about global language delay or a speech problem, especially when a play therapist does not speak a child's mother tongue and thus is unable to assess the child's communication skills in the mother tongue. It is also important to refrain from giving the premature (and possibly misguided) parenting advice of limiting the child's exposure to the mother tongue. Finally, in any play or activity assessment, the play therapist once again needs to be sensitive to the cultural factors affecting the expression of symbolic meaning in play.

Choice of Treatment Modality

Besides individual play therapy and parent consultation, other treatment modalities may be considered. Group play therapy may be an option, as Asian children may feel more comfortable with other youngsters in the playroom. A group format with children from the same or a very similar ethnic background may be particularly helpful. Filial therapy may be another option. Actively engaging parents in learning how to help their children may be an effective way to capitalize on Chinese parents' eagerness to help their own children. The educational component of the filial therapy model may be particularly well received by Chinese parents and may encourage their active participation in the therapy process. Supplementing play therapy with the utilization of community organization resources could be still another way of helping Chinese families. Community resources that are culturally compatible and able to provide services or other assistance in the parents' first language are very helpful (Morrissey, 1997). In particular, Chinese parents are likely to find it easier to connect to an English-speaking play therapist if the therapist has a partnering relationship with professionals (who may not be play therapists but are in the general mental health field) from the Chinese community. Helping Chinese parents to find community resources also enhances social support and increases the chances for successful outcomes of play therapy.

Ethnic Differences between Children and Play Therapists

Will working with a culturally different child be a difficult mission for a play therapist? I would like to share my own experiences in working with children from different ethnic backgrounds during the time when I lived in the United States. The following observations may be helpful for play therapists who are starting to provide services to children from a different culture.

    1. The majority of parents showed their respect for me as a professional. I feel grateful toward those parents from whom I learned my earliest lessons in play therapy. A professional relationship can break the ice between adults of different ethnic backgrounds.

    2. Young children are more likely to cry when they are left alone with a therapist who looks different from most other adults they have come into contact with. I guess that I must have looked strange to my young non-Asian clients, and they felt scared. I accepted the crying while the children took time to feel safe.

    3. Children may be quiet in a relationship with an adult from a different culture. I had more quiet non-Asian clients. From their silent moments, I experienced more fully how play is the language of children. I did not use play and toys to stimulate words from these children. I learned to pay more attention to children's play itself, and thus to gain an understanding of children even when they chose to be quiet in the session.

    4. Even though I came from a different culture, my non-Asian child clients accepted me and developed a good working relationship with me in the playroom. I learned that I could be helpful to clients from a different culture.

    5. In my situation (a Chinese play therapist seeing primarily children of European descent), it was relatively easy to develop an understanding of European American culture, as this was the mainstream culture. When European American play therapists work with clients from an Asian culture, they may need to make an extra effort to educate themselves about the specific culture.

Issues of Countertransference

Cultural countertransference may happen in cross-cultural play therapy situations. That is, in this type of situation, the play therapist's own cultural biases and stereotypes begin to interfere with the therapy process. The focus of therapy may move from the child's presenting issues to the problems that the therapist has projected onto the child and the family. Problems of either positive or negative stereotyping may arise, but in either case, the therapist fails to recognize the child as he or she really is (Johnson, 1993).

It is the therapist's responsibility to maintain awareness of the presence of cultural and other forms of countertransference, and to take appropriate steps to alleviate the situation. Many of these manifestations are best handled in supervision or in discussion with colleagues. There are times when even the most culturally sensitive play therapist may need to refer a child to another therapist so that the child receives the best care.

CONCLUSION

I remember that once I was frustrated about working with culturally different children and complained to my U.S. play therapy supervisor, "I don't understand what the child says." My supervisor smiled and told me wisely, "I don't understand what my child client says sometimes!" Then we laughed together. I laughed because I suddenly realized that I was caught up with my own limitations—the language and culture barriers. I have learned not to waste energy in worrying about my limitations, but rather to spend time expanding my strengths. Now I have students in Taiwan seeing children who speak the same language and complaining to me that they do not understand their child clients' words. I turn this problem back to them and facilitate them in thinking about their real barriers—being afraid of not knowing how to communicate with kids.

Working with an Asian child will be challenging, but not difficult or impossible, if a non-Asian play therapist is willing to learn more about the child's culture and make an extra effort to communicate respect for the child and family. Living in a multicultural context in the United States, with different cultural perspectives, can be truly complementary and enriching if we all embrace a tolerant attitude. By striving for cultural sensitivity and by seeking additional learning opportunities, experiences, and supervision, a therapist will not only be prepared to work with children from different cultures, but will also be part of the movement to promote a vibrant, culturally diverse society in general.

REFERENCES

Csikszentmihalyi, M. (1997). *Finding flow: The psychology of engagement with everyday life*. New York: Basic Books.

Dwivedi, K. N. (1999). *Meeting the needs of ethnic minority children* [Online]. Retrieved from http://www.priory.com/psych/chneeds.htm

Glover, G. (2001). Cultural considerations in play therapy. In G. Landreth (Ed.), *Innovations in play therapy: Issues, process, and special populations* (pp. 31–42). Philadelphia: Brunner-Routledge.

Hall, E. T. (1977). *Beyond culture.* Garden City, NY: Anchor Press.

Huang, G. (1993). *Beyond culture: Communicating with Asian American children* (ERIC Digest No. 94). New York: ERIC Clearinghouse on Urban Education.

Johnson, M. (1993). A culturally sensitive approach to therapy with children. In C. Brems (Ed.), *A comprehensive guide to child psychotherapy* (pp. 68–93). Boston: Allyn & Bacon.

Kao, S.-C., & Landreth, G. (2001). Play therapy with Chinese children: Needed modifications. In G. Landreth (Ed.), *Innovations in play therapy: Issues, process, and special populations* (pp. 43–50). Philadelphia: Brunner-Routledge.

Kleinman, A., & Good, B. J. (1985). *Culture and depression.* Berkeley: University of California Press.

Kong, (1985). Counseling Chinese immigrants: Issues and answers. In R. J. Samuto & A. Wolfgang (Eds.), *Intercultural counseling and assessment: Global perspectives.* Toronto: Hogrefe.

Kottman, T. (2001). *Play therapy: Basics and beyond.* Alexandria, VA: American Counseling Association.

Kuo, C. (1992). *Children play.* Taipei: Young-Chi.

Landreth, G. (1991). *Play therapy: The art of the relationship.* Muncie, IN: Accelerated Development.

Lee, A. (1989). A socio-cultural framework for the assessment of Chinese children with special needs. *Topics in Language Disorders, 9*(3), 38–44.

Lee, G., & Childress, M. (1999). Promising practices: Playing Korean ethnic games to promote multicultural awareness. *Multicultural Education, 6*(3), 33–35.

Manery, G. (2000). *Theraplay with Asian-Canadian families: Practical and theoretical considerations* [Online]. Retrieved from http://www.therapy.org/articles/sum00_pg2.htm

Matsuda, M. (1989). Working with Asian parents: Some communication strategies. *Topics in Language Disorders, 9*(3), 45–53.

Morrissey, M. (1997). The invisible minority: Counseling Asian Americans. *Counseling Today Online.* Retrieved from http://www.counseling.org/ctonline

Nemiroff, M., & Annunziata, J. (1990). *A child's first book about play therapy.* Washington, DC: American Psychological Association.

Pagani-Tousignant, C. (1992). *Breaking the rules: Counseling ethnic minorities.* Minneapolis, MN: Johnson Institute.

Shen, W., & Mo, W. (1990). *Reaching out to their cultures: Building communication with Asian American families.* (ERIC Document Reproduction Service No. ED 351 435)

Sue, D. W., & Sue, D. (2002). *Counseling the culturally diverse: Theory and practice* (4th ed.). New York: Wiley.

Vardell, M. (1996). *Counseling the Asian American client* [Online]. Retrieved from http://www.therapistweb.net/asianamhandout.htm

Appendix

❧

Multicultural Play
Therapy Resources

ATHENA A. DREWES

Play therapy allows a child to utilize play materials to assist in the healing process. It is essential for the play therapist to make sure that the toys available are appropriate and reflect cultural diversity. Be sure the playroom or office has the necessary materials for working with multicultural clients and families. Materials that are highly structured, are stereotyped, or promote antisocial or competitive behavior should be avoided. In order to be sure that the materials being used meet the needs of each client, and do not offend the client or family, I recommend inviting the parent or guardian into the playroom to view what is there. It is also important to encourage the parent/guardian to educate the therapist about the family's cultural and personal metaphors, meanings, beliefs, and religious views; the family's home country (or countries), and trips family members may have taken to see relatives there; and the language(s) spoken in the family. Sensitivity to the images in the playroom is essential, as well as to those in the waiting area and office; no therapist will want to offend clients by inadvertently including something viewed as taboo, or considered bad luck or evil.

SETTING UP THE ENVIRONMENT

The therapist might want to consider hanging paintings, prints, and photos by artists of various cultures that reflect the populations served. Rugs and other textiles, as well as sculptures, pottery, baskets, and other artifacts, can also be displayed (Glover, 1999).

ART AND CRAFT SUPPLIES

Art and craft supplies should definitely include materials that reflect the various cultures of child clients and how each culture may view use of play and play therapy. For example, "in light of the non-verbal communication of affective material typical of Japanese American families, an assessment process using art activities rather than play activities could serve to better inform the therapist" (Hinman, 2002, p. 112). Examples of such items are origami paper for folding, rice paper for painting, and red clay for modeling. Various scraps of imported cloth, leather scraps, and beads and feathers (Glover, 1999) can be used for making collages or creating any number of different projects. Paper reflecting various skin tones should also be included.

Crayola (http://www.crayola.com/store; 1-800-CRAYOLA) has come out with pencils, markers, and crayons that reflect multicultural skin tones. Such materials allow children to make drawings that truly reflect their own families and themselves. These products include 16-count Multicultural Crayons, 8-count Multicultural Colored Pencils, and 8-count Large Multicultural Crayons (thick crayons for little hands). Crayola has described these items as providing "an assortment of hues that gives a child a realistic palette to color the people of the world."

S&S Worldwide (http://www.ssww.com; 1-800-243-9232) has numerous multicultural art and craft supplies. Highlights include Multicultural Washable Markers, Pacon Multicultural Construction Paper, and a Multicultural Bulk Pack (which includes precut people shapes, and many other products); several types of origami paper and ethnic fabric design paper; and Native American Design Impressions for making various symbols in clay.

BOARD GAMES

Games from various cultures may be difficult to find, but these should be included in the therapy room whenever possible. *Mancala*, an African game recently popularized in the United States, is now available at most toy stores. Bilingual games, however, may be difficult to find. *Loteria*, a game from Mexico, is similar to bingo but uses pictures instead of numbers, and may be more familiar than bingo to Mexican parents or grandparents (Martinez & Valdez, 1992).

Marco Products, Inc. (http://www.marcoproducts.com; 1-800-448-2197) carries a game called Multicultural Bingo by Maryann Hudgins, which explores the contributions made by five ethnic groups: African American, Asian American, European American, Hispanic American, and Native American. The game covers holidays, prominent figures, foods, ceremonies, and art contributions of these groups. It is designed for grades 1–6, and any number can play.

BOOKS

The inclusion of books and stories that represent the different cultural groups will be helpful for all the children seen. The children will be able to learn to appreciate each other's diverse backgrounds as well as their own. Books that feature various cultural folktales and heroes should be included. Coloring books of African, Asian, Hispanic, and Native American life and legends are also useful to have in both the waiting room and the therapy room (Martinez & Valdez, 1992).

An excellent resource for books is The Self-Esteem Shop, 32839 Woodward Avenue, Royal Oak, MI 48073 (1-800-251-8336 or http://www.selfesteemshop. com). Its catalog is neatly broken down into categories, and owner DeAnne Ginns-Gruenberg is extremely helpful in recommending titles for any topic or child you are thinking of. Amazon.com http://www.amazon.com) offers online purchasing, as do many other large book distributors.

The following subsections highlight noteworthy children's books about youngsters of various ethnicities, from the ever-expanding selection available.

African American

- *Afro-Bets Kids: I'm Gonna Be!* by Wade Hudson, 1992, Just Us Books. ISBN 0940975408. (Also available as e-book; iPicture Books. ISBN B00005TNT7. African American children explore what they might grow up to become, using the various African American role models described in the story. Additional series of Afro-Bets Kids books are available now.

- *Amazing Grace* by Mary Hoffman and Caroline Binch, 1991, Scott, Foresman. ISBN 0803710402. Grace wants to play the role of Peter Pan in the school production. Her classmates object, preferring a white male to a black female. But Grace perseveres, proving to everyone that she can accomplish anything. Sequels to this book are also available.

- *Black like Kyra, White like Me* by Judith Vigna, 1996, Albert Whitman. ISBN 0807507792. Kyra and Christy are best friends, but when Kyra moves to the neighborhood, she and her family encounter racism and vandalism.

- *Bright Eyes, Brown Skin* by Cheryl Willis Hudson and Bernette G. Ford, 1996, Sundance Pubns (paperback). ISBN 9996136825. Story of how four African American preschool children feel good about who they are and how they look.

- *Grandpa, Is Everything Black Bad?* by Sandy Lynne Holman, 1998, Culture Co Op. ISBN 0964465515. An illustrated story of an African American boy who comes to appreciate his dark skin by learning about his African heritage from his grandfather.

- *I Love My Hair!* by Natasha Tarpley, 1998, Megan Tingley. ISBN 0316522759. An African American girl loves it when her mother brushes her hair, and she enjoys the different styles she can try.

- *Jamaica and the Substitute Teacher* by Juanita Havill, 2001, Houghton Mifflin. ISBN 0618152423. Latest in a series about Jamaica, an African American girl whose teacher helps her learn that she does not have to be perfect to be special.
- *Nappy Hair* by Carolivia Herron, 1998, Random House (reprint). ISBN 0679894454. Various African American people at a backyard picnic offer their comments on a young girl's tightly curled, "nappy" hair. Colorful, culturally appropriate drawings and use of language.
- *Read for Me, Mama* by Vashanti Rahaman, 1997, Boyds Mills. ISBN 1563973138. Joseph, an African American boy, discovers his mother's illiteracy and helps her learn to read.
- *Sosu's Call* by Meshack Asare, 2002, Cranky Nell Books. ISBN 1929132212. When a great storm threatens, Sosu, an African boy who is unable to walk, joins his dog, Fusa, in helping save their village.
- *The Color of Us* by Karen Katz, 2002, Henry Holt. ISBN 0805071636. Lena wants to color a picture of herself, and learns that not all browns are the same.
- *Words by Heart* by Ouida Sebestyen, 1997, Yearling Books. ISBN 044041346X. Vowing to gain her father's approval and her white classmates' respect by winning a Bible-quoting contest, Lena (not the same Lena as in the preceding book) is horrified when success brings violence and death to her home.

Asian American

- *Allison* by Allen Say, 1997, Houghton Mifflin. ISBN 039585895X. An Asian child begins to realize that she is different from her parents. The book focuses on families, adoption, and the search for belonging.
- *Baseball Saved Us*, by Ken Mochezuki, 1995, Lee & Low Books. ISBN 1880000199. Story of a Japanese American boy and his family in a U.S. internment camp during World War II, and how baseball helped ease the time.
- *Char Siu Bao Boy* by Sandra Yamate, 2000, Polychrome. ISBN 1879965194. Charlie loves *char siu bao* and eats it every day, but his friends think it is awful.
- *Dear Juno*, by Soyung Pak, 2001, Puffin. ISBN 0142300179. A Korean American boy and his grandmother in Korea correspond and transcend language barriers.
- *Dumpling Soup* by Jama Kim Rattigan, 1998, Megan Tingley (reprint). ISBN 0316730475. A Korean family living on a Hawaiian island has a tradition of making dumplings for New Year's.
- *Grandfather's Journey* by Allen Say, 1993, Houghton Mifflin. ISBN 0395570352. A story of Japanese immigration and acculturation.
- *I Love You Like Crazy Cakes* by Rose Lewis, 2000, Little, Brown. ISBN 0316525383. A book about Chinese children and adoption.
- *Kids Like Me in China* by Ying Ying Fry, Amy Klatzkin, and Brian Boyd, 2001, Yeong & Yeong. ISBN 0963847260. Adoption and China as seen through the eyes of Ying Ying, a real-life 8-year-old.

- *Moonbeams, Dumplings and Dragon Boats: A Treasury of Chinese Holiday Tales, Activities and Recipes* by Nina Simonds and Leslie Swartz, 2002, Gulliver Books. ISBN 0152019839. A book about Chinese holidays, with brief background descriptions, recipes, crafts and legends.
- *Tea with Milk* by Allen Say, 1999, Houghton Mifflin. ISBN 0395904951. A story about the author's mother, a Japanese girl born in America who had to adapt to Japan as a teenager when her family returned there.
- *Who Belongs Here?* by Margy Burns Knight and Anne Sibley O'Brien, 1993, Tilbury House. ISBN 0884481107. Nary escapes Cambodia and comes to America only to encounter prejudice.

Hispanic

- *A Day's Work* by Eve Bunting, 1997, Houghton Mifflin. ISBN 0395845181. Immigration story about the reversal of roles when a Mexican American boy acts as interpreter for his newly arrived grandfather.
- *Going Home* by Eve Bunting, 1998, Harper Trophy. ISBN 0064435091. A portrait of a migrant Mexican family leaving home for America.
- *My Very Own Room/Mi Propio Cuarito* by Amanda Irma Perez, 2000, Children's Book Press. ISBN 0892391642. The story of a Mexican American girl's search for her own space in an overflowing house, told in both English and Spanish.
- *Salsa Stories* by Lulu Delacre, 2000, Scholastic. ISBN 0590631187. Stories of holidays from Guatemala, Puerto Rico, Mexico, Peru, and Argentina.
- *The Latino Holiday Book: From Cinco de Mayo to Dia de los Muertos: The Celebrations and Traditions of Hispanic-Americans* by Valerie Menard, 2000, Diane Publishing (paperback). ISBN 0756765714. A full year of holidays covering Mexican, Cuban, and Puerto Rican heritage.
- *The Most Beautiful Place in the World* by Ann Cameron, 1993, Yearling Books. ISBN 0394804244. The trials and tribulations of 7-year-old Juan in Guatemala, who is abandoned by his mother.
- *Too Many Tamales* by Gary Soto, 1996, Puffin. ISBN 0698114124. The story of a Christmas celebration in South America.
- *We Are a Rainbow* by Nancy Maria Grande Tabor, 1997, Charlesbridge. ISBN 0881064173. Mexican children move to the United States and compare the differences and similarities of cultures.

Native American

- *Bluebonnet Girl* by Michael Lind, 2003, Henry Holt. ISBN 0805065733. Comanche legend of how Texas became known as the Bluebonnet State.
- *Everybody Needs a Rock* by Byrd Baylor, 1985, Scott, Foresman. ISBN 0689710518. According to Native American lore, everybody needs a rock as a friend. The books gives 10 rules for finding the perfect rock.

• *Fire in Her Hair: A Story of Friendship* by D. Kelley Steele, 2002, Hidden Path. ISBN 097115340X. The story of a girl's courage to stand up to taunts.

• *Home to Medicine Mountain* by Chiori Santiago, 2002, Children's Book Press. ISBN 0892391766. A true story from the 1930s, of children sent to spend a year in a strict government residential school separated from Native American culture and family.

• *Mama, Do You Love Me?* by Barbara M. Joosse, 1998, Chronicle Books. ISBN 0811821315. Timeless story about a daughter's attempt to find the limit of her mother's love. Beautiful illustrations of Alaska and Eskimo family life.

• *Raven: A Trickster Tale from the Pacific Northwest* by Gerald McDermott, 1993, Harcourt. ISBN 0152656618. A retelling of the Native American tale describing the birth of the sun.

Multicultural

• *All the Colors We Are: The Story of How We Get Our Skin Color* by Katie Kissinger, 1997, Redleaf Press. ISBN 0934140804. Children learn how we get our skin color, and see pictures of different-colored people.

• *Black Is Brown Is Tan* by Arnold Adoff, 2002, Armistad Press. ISBN 0060287764. Illustrated book in verse about a family with a brown-skinned mother, a light-skinned father, and their two children, along with various relatives.

• *Come and Abide (We Are All the Same Inside)* by Timothy Bellavia and Randi Cannata's 4th Grade T.A.G. @ P.S. 175Q, District 28—N.Y.C., 2002, Tolerance in Multi-Media Education (T.I.M.M.-E). ISBN 0971823200. A book that helps young learners understand tolerance while exploring various aspects of diversity.

• *Different Just Like Me* by Lori Mitchell, 2001, Charlesbridge. ISBN 1570914907. Illustrated story about a young girl who notices that, like the flowers in Grammie's garden, people who are different from one another also share many qualities, and it's okay to like them all the same.

• *Everybody Has Feelings/Todos Tenemos Sentimientos: The Moods of Children* by Charles E. Avery, 1998 (reprint), Gryphon House. ISBN 0876591977. Photographs of multicultural children, with text in both English and Spanish exploring a wide range of human emotions.

• *If the World Were Blind ...* by Karen Gedig Burnett, 2001, GR. ISBN 0966853040. When Jackson asks his grandfather why people have trouble getting along, it makes them think about how things might be better if we all looked past physical attributes to see the person underneath.

• *It's Okay to Be Me!* by Ja'Nitta Marbury, 2001, Shades of Me. ISBN 097183071. Various children introduce their races, ethnicities, and cultures, affirming their individual identities.

• *Peace in Our Land: Children Celebrating Diversity* by Bunny Hull and Synthia Saint James, 2002, Brassheart. ISBN 0967376297. A book that teaches children to respect diversity—racial, cultural, physical, and religious.

- *To Be a Kid* by Maya Ajmera and John D. Ivanko, 2000, Charlesbridge. ISBN 088106842X. Text and photographs from countries around the world illustrate some of the activities children everywhere have in common.
- *We All Have a Heritage* by Sandy Lynne Holman, 2002, Culture Co Op. ISBN 0964465523. An illustrated story of children from diverse cultural backgrounds who learn and celebrate the facts that we all have a heritage and we have a lot in common.

DRAMATIC PLAY AREA AND RESOURCES

As in most playrooms, items that reflect nurturing themes for dramatic play should be included, such as dishes, cooking utensils, and food items from various cultures (along with items from the dominant culture). The therapist can obtain some culturally related items inexpensively from such places as Dollar Stores, which carry merchandise appropriate to the communities in which they are located; other items can be purchased from local merchants within these communities (e.g., at Asian grocery stores). In this way, the play therapist not only can pick up items for the playroom but can also learn more about each community's activities and people. "Items that reflect diverse cultures include tea boxes, tea tins, canned foods, cardboard food containers, plastic bottles, plastic play food . . . baskets, gourds, mesh bags and pottery" (Glover, 1999, p. 290). Such items as a strainer, ladle, wok, tortilla press, tea ball, frying pan, kettle, wooden spoons, graters, whisk, rice bowl, wooden bowls and plates, and chopsticks can also be included (Glover, 1999).

Childcraft (http://www.childcraft.com) sells a 63-piece Multicultural Food Set that represents food and utensils from around the world, such as egg rolls, sushi, bamboo steamer, tacos, kiwi, and more. They also have Play Food in a Basket (23 pieces of canned items, frozen food boxes, plastic bottles, and boxes), as well as an Aluminum Cooking Set (with a realistic strainer, ladle, tea kettle, pots, and pans).

In addition to nurturing items, action figures for dramatic play should also be included for use by girls and boys. For example, miniatures of Ninja figures, available in most dollar stores, as well as GI Joe dolls with ethnic features, should be included.

DOLLS

Dolls of all sizes, shapes, and ages can now be purchased in different skin colors, as well as with realistic facial characteristics, different hair colors or styles, and culturally appropriate clothing. Barbie dolls now come in various skin tones and features. Several companies and catalogs have multicultural baby dolls, as well as dollhouse families. Scraps of batik fabric, *kente* cloth, or other colorful woven fabric can also be used as doll blankets or even for dress-up.

Childcraft (http://www.childcraft.com) has a wide and varied assortment of multicultural dolls, only some of which are described here. Infant/Toddler Washable Soft Baby Dolls are 10" rag dolls that come in various skin tones. Also available are 13" and 16" boy and girl vinyl dolls in Asian, black, white, and Hispanic skin tones and features, as well as several types of soft-body baby dolls in black and white skin tones. Childcraft also has boy and girl Special Needs Dolls in Hispanic, black, Asian, and white skin tones and features, with accessories such as crutches and a wheelchair that can be purchased separately. Turn-Me-Around Expressions Dolls are 14" huggable boy and girl dolls with a happy face on one side of the head and a sad face on the other; again, these are available in Asian, black, white, and Hispanic skin tones and features. The Poseable Family sets have jointed arms, legs, heads, and hips; they include grandparents, parents, boy, and girl in black and white skin tones, and can be used in dollhouse play. Pretend-Play dolls are 5" realistically detailed, solid vinyl, free-standing family sets (grandparents, parents, boy, girl, younger girl, and baby boy) in black, white, Asian, and Hispanic skin tones and features. Wooden Dollhouse Families (parents, boy, and girl) are dressed in fabric clothes and come in white, black, Hispanic, and Asian skin tones and features.

Childswork/Childsplay (http://www.childswork.com; 1-800-962-1141) carries a Wooden Doll House and people in white and black skin tones.

Manhattan Toy (http://www.manhattantoy.com) makes the Groovy Girls series of 13" soft fabric girl (and some boy) dolls in various skin tones with ethnically appropriate hair.

Rose Play Therapy Toys (http://www.roseplaytherapy.com; 1-800-713-2252) has anatomically detailed boy and girl baby dolls in white and black skin tones, as well as 14" dolls in white, black, and Hispanic skin tones.

The Self-Esteem Shop (http://www.selfesteemshop.com; 1-800-251-8336) offers Anatomically Correct Dolls in Hispanic, Caucasian (i.e., European American), and African American skin tones; Bendable Dollhouse Families for dollhouse play in Asian, African American, Hispanic, and Caucasian family sets multicultural playmobil people; and Worry Dolls, six small dolls in a box (the box describes a Native American/indigenous people's legend that when you have troubles, you should share them with one of the dolls before going to sleep—the doll will solve the troubles for you, helping you to sleep peacefully).

Ty (http://www.ty.com) makes a Beanie Baby series (Teenie Beanie Boppers) with boys and girls in various sizes and skin tones, and with Afros or braided hair.

Western Psychological Services: Creative Therapy Store (http://www.creativetherapystore.com; 1-800-648-8857) has Real People Dolls (anatomical dolls) in black, brown, and white skin tones; Pose and Play Doll *Families* for dollhouse use in black, white, and Hispanic sets; and DUPLO World People, which are 24 culturally diverse figures (representing four ethnic groups and three generations) that can be used alone, with a dollhouse, or with the DUPLO Home.

PUPPETS

There is a wide array of multicultural puppets on the market, from finger size on up, dressed to reflect all types of professions and ages.

Childcraft (http://www.childcraft.com) has Multicultural Career Puppets in all plastic; Career Puppets in all cloth; Pro-Diversity Puppets in fabric, representing various occupations; a Hug and Hold Doll/Puppets Set of four 13½" figures with different skin tones; and Family Puppet Sets (parents, boy, girl, and baby; adults are 11") in black, white, Asian, and Hispanic skin tones.

Childswork/Childsplay (http://www.childswork.com; 1-800-962-1141) carries Our Favorite Puppets, realistic hand puppets with plastic heads in Asian, Hispanic, Caucasian, and African American family groups (man, woman, boy, girl, and baby). It also has Multiethnic Families, dollhouse-sized puppets in Caucasian, African American, Hispanic, and Asian family groups with rubber bodies and removable cloth clothing.

Manhattan Toy (http://www.manhattantoy.com) has a doctor hand puppet in fabric with black skin tone, as well as Global Dance Finger Puppets, which are four puppets in four ethnic outfits (Hawaiian, Asian, Middle Eastern, and Russian).

Marco Products, Inc. (http://www.marcoproducts.com; 1-800-448-2197) has Family Puppet Sets (man, woman, boy, girl, and baby) in African American, Asian American, Hispanic, and Caucasian skin tones. It also has a set of seven Community Helper Puppets (postal worker, doctor, firefighter, police officer, construction worker, teacher, nurse) with four having black and three white skin tones.

Rose Play Therapy Toys (http://www.roseplaytherapy.com; 1-800-713-2252) has 14" hand puppets of a man and woman with white and black skin tones, and a five-piece puppet set with rubber/plastic heads in black, Hispanic, and white skin tones.

The Self-Esteem Shop (http://www.selfesteemshop.com; 1-800-251-8336) has Interchangeable People Puppets with gender-neutral bodies that children can add clothing, legs, and hair to. They come in Caucasian, African American, or Hispanic skin tones.

SANDTRAY MINIATURES

Anna's Toy Depot (http://www.annastoydepot.com; 1-888-227-9169) has a wide variety of miniatures. These include religious figures and symbols; landscape figures; and various human figurines (including Teen Dancers; a black, white, and Hispanic Bride and Groom; and a white Priest and black Preacher). Dollhouse figures (which can also be used in the sandtray) include Bendable Families (parents, girl, and baby boy) in black, white, and Hispanic skin tones, with additional Bendable Children and Grandparents available; a set of multicultural Community Members, with white, black, Hispanic, and Asian skin tones and features; and black, white, Hispanic, and Asian family members (nonbendable).

Rose Play Therapy Toys (http://www.roseplaytherapy.com; 1-800-713-2252) carries a variety of multicultural human figures and religious symbols. The human figures include an eight-piece Pretend Play Family (grandparents, man, woman, boy, girl, toddler boy, and toddler girl) in black and white skin tones; three varieties of smaller dollhouse five-piece family sets in black, white, and Hispanic skin tones; individual 3½" girl and boy dolls in white and black skin tones; white and black man and woman bridal figures; and white and black sleeping boy and girl babies.

MISCELLANEOUS

Ethnic music from different cultures can be used during sessions or played as background music in a waiting room. The inclusion of a globe or maps of the world or different countries can help spark discussion during therapy about emigration and immigration, or can help clarify a family's points of origin (Martinez & Valdez, 1992).

A good resource for obtaining ethnic baskets, rugs, toys, books, and items for your office is through catalogs of nonprofit agencies that help to market the wares and crafts of indigenous peoples in an effort to financially support their economy. Below are a few organizations that have items that would be useful for play therapists.

Christian Children's Fund Global Crafts (http://www. christianchildrens fund.org; 1-800-776-6767) has an assortment of items such as toys, animals, figures, dolls, baskets, and musical instruments from indigenous peoples around the world.

SERRV International (http://www.serrv.org; 1-800-422-5915) sells an assortment of handmade toys and crafts, dolls, puppets, rugs, and instruments from Mexico, India, Africa, South America, and the Philippines.

The Southwest Indian Foundation (http://www.southwestindian.com; 1-505-863-4037) assists Navajo, Hopi, and Zuni reservation tribes in the Southwest by selling an assortment of items including kachinas, dolls, books, pottery, textiles, and toys. They have a GI Joe: Navajo Code Talker doll with ethnic skin tones and features and that speaks seven different phrases in both Navajo and English. They also have a Northern Cheyenne action figure and Apache War Leader action figure with detailed features, face paint, and clothing.

UNICEF (http://www.unicefusa.org; 1-800-553-1200) has beautifully drawn storybooks and coloring books about various countries of the world. It also has *A Life Like Mine*, which is a book with colorful photographs of children throughout the world, and the commonalties through the challenges they face and their passion for life. *Children Just Like Me* is a colorfully photographed book of children around the world and the cultural diversity of festivals and holidays.

REFERENCES

Glover, G. (1999). Multicultural considerations in group play therapy. In D. S. Sweeney & L. E. Homeyer (Eds.), *The handbook of group play therapy* (pp. 278–295). San Francisco: Jossey-Bass.

Hinman, C. (2003). Multicultural considerations in the delivery of play therapy services. *International Journal of Play Therapy, 12*(2), 107–122.

Martinez, K. J., & Valdez, D. M. (1992). Cultural considerations in play therapy with Hispanic children. In L. A. Vargas & J. D. Koss-Chioino (Eds.), *Working with culture* (pp. 85–102). San Francisco: Jossey-Bass.

Index

Page numbers followed by an *f* indicate figure, *n* indicate note.

UNIVERSITY OF MAINE AT AUGUSTA

3 2304 00085842 1

DEMCO

OCT   4 2006